INTERVENTIONAL CARDIOLOGY CLINICS

www.interventional.theclinics.com

Editor-in-Chief

MARVIN H. ENG

Intracoronary Imaging and Its Use in Interventional Cardiology

April 2023 • Volume 12 • Number 2

Editor

YASUHIRO HONDA

ELSEVIER

1600 John F. Kennedy Boulevard • Suite 1800 • Philadelphia, Pennsylvania, 19103-2899

http://www.theclinics.com

INTERVENTIONAL CARDIOLOGY CLINICS Volume 12, Number 2
April 2023 ISSN 2211-7458, ISBN-13: 978-0-323-93997-3

Editor: Joanna Gascoine
Developmental Editor: Arlene B. Campos

Interventional Cardiology Clinics (ISSN 2211-7458) is published quarterly by Elsevier Inc., 360 Park Avenue South, New York, NY 10010-1710. Months of issue are January, April, July, and October. Subscription prices are USD 217 per year for US individuals, USD 570 for US institutions, USD 100 per year for US students, USD 217 per year for Canadian individuals, USD 679 for Canadian institutions, USD 100 per year for Canadian students, USD 308 per year for international individuals, USD 679 for international institutions, and USD 150 per year for international students. To receive student/resident rate, orders must be accompanied by name of affiliated institution, date of term, and the *signature* of program/residency coordinator on institution letterhead. Orders will be billed at individual rate until proof of status is received. Foreign air speed delivery is included in all *Clinics* subscription prices. All prices are subject to change without notice. **POSTMASTER:** Send address changes to *Interventional Cardiology Clinics*, Elsevier Health Sciences Division, Subscription Customer Service, 3251 Riverport Lane, Maryland Heights, MO 63043. **Customer Service: Telephone: 1-800-654-2452** (U.S. and Canada); **1-314-447-8871** (outside U.S. and Canada). **Fax: 1-314-447-8029. E-mail: journalscustomerservice-usa@elsevier.com (for print support); journalsonlinesupport-usa@elsevier.com (for online support).**

Reprints. For copies of 100 or more of articles in this publication, please contact the Commercial Reprints Department, Elsevier Inc., 360 Park Avenue South, New York, NY 10010-1710. Tel.: 212-633-3874; Fax: 212-633-3820; E-mail: reprints@elsevier.com.

CONTRIBUTORS

CONSULTING EDITOR

MARVIN H. ENG, MD
Structural Heart Program Medical Director,
Structural Heart Disease Fellowship Director,
Director of Cardiovascular Quality, Banner
University Medical Center, Phoenix,
Arizona, USA

EDITOR

YASUHIRO HONDA, MD, FACC, FAHA
Clinical Professor of Medicine, Director of
Cardiovascular Core Analysis Laboratory,
Division of Cardiovascular Medicine, Stanford
Cardiovascular Institute, Stanford University
School of Medicine, Stanford, California, USA

AUTHORS

ARSALAN ABU-MUCH, MD
Cardiovascular Research Foundation, New
York, New York, USA

JUNYA AKO, MD
Department of Cardiovascular Medicine,
Kitasato University School of Medicine,
Kanagawa, Japan

ZIAD A. ALI, MD, DPhil
Department of Cardiology, St. Francis
Hospital, Roslyn, New York, USA;
Cardiovascular Research Foundation, New
York, New York, USA

RONALD D. BASS, BA
School of Medicine, Georgetown University,
Washington DC, USA

CHRISTOS V. BOURANTAS, MD, PhD
Department of Cardiology, Barts Heart
Centre, Barts Health NHS Trust, Institute of
Cardiovascular Science, University College
London, London, United Kingdom

KAREN CHAU, BS
Department of Cardiology, St. Francis
Hospital, Roslyn, New York, USA

BRIAN COURTNEY, MD
Schulich Heart Program, Sunnybrook Research
Institute, University of Toronto, Toronto,
Ontario, Canada

ALI DAKROUB, MD
Department of Cardiology, St. Francis
Hospital, Roslyn, New York, USA

HECTOR M. GARCIA-GARCIA, MD, PhD
Professor, Interventional Cardiology, MedStar
Washington Hospital Center, Washington,
DC, USA

SCOT GARG, MD, PhD
Department of Cardiology, Royal
Blackburn Hospital, Blackburn, United
Kingdom

TAKEHIRO HASHIKATA, MD
Department of Cardiovascular Medicine,
Kitasato University School of Medicine,
Kanagawa, Japan

KIYOSHI HIBI, MD, PhD
Division of Cardiology, Yokohama City
University Medical Center

MYEONG-KI HONG, MD
Severance Hospital, Yonsei University College
of Medicine, Seoul, South Korea

JIAYUE HUANG, MSc
Department of Cardiology, National
University of Ireland, Galway (NUIG), Galway,
Ireland

SHINJI INABA, MD, PhD
Department of Cardiology, Pulmonology, Hypertension and Nephrology, Ehime University Graduate School of Medicine, Toon, Ehime, Japan

ALLEN JEREMIAS, MD, MSc
Department of Cardiology, St. Francis Hospital, Roslyn, New York, USA; Cardiovascular Research Foundation, New York, New York, USA

SHIGETAKA KAGEYAMA, MD
Department of Cardiology, National University of Ireland, Galway (NUIG), Galway, Ireland

RYO KAMEDA, MD
Department of Cardiovascular Medicine, Kitasato University School of Medicine, Kanagawa, Japan

KEYVAN KARIMI GALOUGAHI, MD, PhD
Department of Cardiology, St. Francis Hospital, Roslyn, New York, USA

NOZOMI KOTOKU, MD
Department of Cardiology, National University of Ireland, Galway (NUIG), Galway, Ireland

TAKASHI KUBO, MD
Director, Department of Cardiovascular Medicine, Naga Municipal Hospital, Wakayama, Japan

YONG-JOON LEE, MD
Severance Hospital, Yonsei University College of Medicine, Seoul, South Korea

RYAN D. MADDER, MD
Frederik Meijer Heart and Vascular Institute, Spectrum Health, Grand Rapids, Grand Rapids, Michigan, USA

AKIKO MAEHARA, MD
Cardiovascular Research Foundation, New York, New York, USA

SHINICHIRO MASUDA, MD
Department of Cardiology, National University of Ireland, Galway (NUIG), Galway, Ireland

MITSUAKI MATSUMURA, BS
Cardiovascular Research Foundation, New York, New York, USA

GARY S. MINTZ, MD
Cardiovascular Research Foundation, New York, New York, USA

ISAO MORI, MS
Terumo Corporation, Tokyo, Japan

KAI NINOMIYA, MD
Department of Cardiology, National University of Ireland, Galway (NUIG), Galway, Ireland

KENSUKE NISHIMIYA, MD, PhD
Department of Cardiovascular Medicine, Tohoku University Graduate School of Medicine, Sendai, Miyagi, Japan

KOICHI NODE, MD, PhD
Department of Cardiovascular Medicine, Saga University, Saga, Japan

KOZO OKADA, MD, PhD
Division of Cardiology, Yokohama City University Medical Center

TAKAYUKI OKAMURA, MD, PhD
Division of Cardiology, Department of Medicine and Clinical Science, Yamaguchi University Graduate School of Medicine, Yamaguchi, Japan

YOSHINOBU ONUMA, MD, PhD
Department of Cardiology, Professor of Interventional Cardiology, National University of Ireland, Galway (NUIG), Galway, Ireland

HIROMASA OTAKE, MD, PhD, FACC
Division of Cardiovascular Medicine, Department of Internal Medicine, Kobe University Graduate School of Medicine, Kobe, Hyogo, Japan

MALAV J. PARIKH, MD
Frederik Meijer Heart and Vascular Institute, Spectrum Health, Grand Rapids, Grand Rapids, Michigan, USA

RUSHI V. PARIKH, MD
Division of Cardiology, University of California, Los Angeles, Los Angeles, California, USA

JOSEPH PHILLIPS, BS, MS
University of Iowa Hospitals and Clinics, Iowa City, Iowa, USA

RADHIKA K. PODUVAL, PhD
Wellman Center for Photomedicine, Massachusetts General Hospital, Harvard Medical School, Boston, Massachusetts, USA

JORGE SANZ SÁNCHEZ, MD, PhD
Hospital Universitari I Politecnic La Fe, Valencia, Spain; Centro de Investigación Biomedica en Red (CIBERCV), Madrid, Spain

FUMIYASU SEIKE, MD, PhD
Department of Cardiology, Pulmonology, Hypertension and Nephrology, Ehime University Graduate School of Medicine, Toon, Ehime, Japan

PATRICK W. SERRUYS, MD, PhD
Department of Cardiology, National University of Ireland, Galway (NUIG), Galway, Ireland

PRITI SHAH, MSC
Infraredx, A Nipro Company, Bedford, Massachusetts, USA

NEGEEN SHAHANDEH, MD
Division of Cardiology, University of California, Los Angeles, Los Angeles, California, USA

FAISAL SHARIF, MD, PhD
Department of Cardiology, National University of Ireland, Galway (NUIG), Galway, Ireland

EVAN S. SHLOFMITZ, DO
Department of Cardiology, St. Francis Hospital, Roslyn, New York, USA

RICHARD A. SHLOFMITZ, MD
Department of Cardiology, St. Francis Hospital, Roslyn, New York, USA

SHINJO SONODA, MD, PhD
Department of Cardiovascular Medicine, Saga University, Saga, Japan

STEPHEN SUM, PhD
Infraredx, A Nipro Company, Bedford, Massachusetts, USA

GUILLERMO J. TEARNEY, MD, PhD
Wellman Center for Photomedicine, Harvard Medical School, Professor, Department of Pathology, Massachusetts General Hospital, Boston, Massachusetts, USA; Harvard-MIT Division of Health Sciences and Technology Division, Cambridge, Massachusetts, USA

SUSAN V. THOMAS, MPH
Department of Cardiology, St. Francis Hospital, Roslyn, New York, USA

RON WAKSMAN, MD
Interventional Cardiology, MedStar Washington Hospital Center, Washington, DC, USA

NICK WEST, MD
Abbott Vascular, Santa Clara, California, USA

OSAMU YAMAGUCHI, MD, PhD
Department of Cardiology, Pulmonology, Hypertension and Nephrology, Ehime University Graduate School of Medicine, Toon, Ehime, Japan

KAZUNORI YASUDA, PhD
Department of Mechanical Engineering, Ehime University Graduate School of Science and Engineering, Matsuyama, Ehime, Japan

CONTENTS

> Vulnerable plaque plays a pivotal role in the pathogenesis of acute coronary syndrome (ACS), being responsible for most ACS. The concept of vulnerable plaque has evolved with advancements in basic and clinical investigations along with developments and rapid expansion of coronary imaging modalities. Intravascular ultrasound (IVUS) is the first widely applied clinical technology with sufficient tissue penetration and enables us to identify vulnerable plaque and comprehensively understand the pathophysiology of ACS. In this review, we summarize current clinical evidence established by IVUS and the recent advancements in our understanding of vulnerable plaque and its role in ACS management.

> Why is intravascular ultrasounography (IVUS) highly encouraged for the practical guidance of percutaneous coronary intervention (PCI)? First reason is to understand the mechanism of revascularization. Even if stenoses look similar in angiography, the pathophysiology could be different in each lesion. Second reason is to anticipate possible complications in advance. With prediction and appropriate preparation, most complications can be avoided or managed calmly when they occur. Third reason is to optimize PCI results with interactive IVUS use during the procedure. All these are essential to maximize the results of revascularization while minimizing acute complications, ultimately leading to improved long-term clinical outcomes.

> The intravascular ultrasound (IVUS)-guided percutaneous coronary intervention (PCI) that was associated with improved post-procedural outcomes and long-term clinical outcomes has shown benefits not only in patients with complex lesions but also with simplex lesions. However, the use of IVUS during PCI remains low; therefore, further prospective, randomized, controlled trials are required to strengthen the recommendations and consequently expand its usage. The aim of this review is to discuss the previous evidences and clinical trials regarding IVUS-guided PCI and to discover the necessity for future studies to broaden its use in the real-world clinical practice.

▶ Video content accompanies this article at http://www.interventional.theclinics.com.

Intravascular ultrasound (IVUS) and optical coherence tomography (OCT) are established intravascular imaging tools for evaluating plaque characteristics and volume, together with guiding percutaneous coronary interventions. The high tissue penetration of IVUS facilitates assessment of the entire vessel wall, whereas the higher resolution of OCT allows detailed assessment of endoluminal structures. A combined IVUS-OCT probe works synergistically, facilitating a greater understanding of de novo coronary artery disease and a better correlation with pathological specimens. In this review, we discuss the rationale and potential roles of the combined IVUS–OCT catheter system.

Optical coherence tomography (OCT) is an intravascular imaging technique that uses near-infrared light. OCT provides high-resolution cross-sectional images of coronary arteries and enables tissue characterization of atherosclerotic plaques. OCT can identify plaque rupture, plaque erosion, and calcified nodule in culprit lesions of acute coronary syndrome. OCT can also detect important morphologic features of vulnerable plaques such as thin fibrous caps, large lipid cores, macrophages accumulation, intraplaque microvasculature, cholesterol crystals, healed plaques, and intraplaque hemorrhage.

Optical coherence tomography (OCT) provides high-resolution imaging of coronary arteries and can be used to optimize percutaneous coronary intervention (PCI). Intracoronary OCT, however, has had limited adoption in clinical practice. Novelty and relative complexity of OCT interpretation compared with the more established intravascular ultrasound, lack of a standardized algorithm for PCI guidance, paucity of data from randomized trials, and lack of rebate for intravascular imaging have contributed to the modest practical adoption of OCT. We provide a practical step-by-step guide on how to use OCT in PCI, including device set-up, simplified image interpretation, and an algorithmic approach for PCI. optimization.

Intracoronary imaging is beneficial to optimize stent implantation and reduce the risk of stent-related complications. Optical coherence tomography (OCT) is an intravascular imaging modality that allows for detailed microstructural evaluation during the percutaneous coronary intervention (PCI). Recently, several large-scale registries, randomized trials, and meta-analyses have shown the superiority of OCT to angiography and noninferiority to IVUS with respect to both acute procedural results and mid-term clinical outcomes. This article summarizes the data supporting the application of OCT-guided PCI to several specific situations, introduces important evidence, and discusses the ongoing controversies and limitations of the current evidence base in the field of OCT-guided PCI.

Optical coherence tomography (OCT) is an imaging modality that is used in a significant number of interventional cardiology procedures. Key structural changes occurring within the vessel wall, including presence of neutrophils, macrophages, monocytes, and vascular smooth muscle cells, are below the resolution of clinical intracoronary OCT. To address this challenge, a new form of OCT with 1 to 2 μm resolution, termed micro-OCT (μOCT), has been developed. This review article summarizes the ability of μOCT technology to visualize coronary microstructures and discusses its clinical implications.

Previous studies have analyzed the efficacy of near-infrared spectroscopy-derived lipid core burden index (LCBI) in quantifying and identifying high-risk plaques and patients at increased risk of future major adverse cardiac outcomes/major adverse cardiovascular and cerebrovascular events. A $maxLCBI_{4mm}$ of 400 or greater seems to be an effective threshold for classifying at-risk plaques. This meta-analysis provides a more precise odds ratio with a narrow standard deviation that can be used to guide future studies.

Intracoronary near-infrared spectroscopy (NIRS) has been extensively validated against the gold standard of histopathology to identify lipid-rich plaque. NIRS is currently in clinical use as a combined multimodality imaging catheter with intravascular ultrasonography. When used before PCI, NIRS has clinical utility in determining the mechanism underlying acute coronary syndromes and can be used to guide stent length selection and identify the risk of periprocedural myocardial infarction. When used after PCI, NIRS can identify vulnerable patients at increased risk of future patient-level cardiovascular events and can detect vulnerable plaques at increased risk of future site-specific coronary events.

Despite advances in the care of heart transplant recipients during the past 5 decades, cardiac allograft vasculopathy (CAV) continues to be a major barrier to long-term survival. The early diagnosis and treatment of CAV is crucial for improving long-term outcomes. Coronary angiography, the current gold standard for CAV screening, has low sensitivity for detecting early CAV. Increasingly, invasive intracoronary imaging modalities that provide a more detailed analysis of vessel anatomy and allow for plaque characterization are being used to detect CAV earlier after transplant and uncover mechanistic insights. Studies validating these emerging imaging platforms are needed before their widespread adoption.

Myocardial bridging (MB) was historically considered a benign structure as most people with MB are clinically asymptomatic. Recently, however, mounting evidence indicates that MB can cause adverse cardiac events owing to arterial systolic compression/diastolic restriction, atherosclerotic plaque progression upstream from MB, and/or vasospastic angina. In MB patients with refractory angina, the optimal treatment strategy should be determined individually based on versatile anatomic and hemodynamical assessments that often require multidisciplinary diagnostic approaches. The present review summarizes the clinical implication and management of MB, highlighting the role of imaging modalities currently available in this arena.

Intravascular imaging (IVI) is clinically useful for assessing the lesion structure and characteristics; however, it is not designed to estimate myocardial ischemia. Several types of IVI-derived fractional flow reserve (FFR) (IVI-derived-FFR) have been developed. The algorithms of IVI-derived-FFR are based on basic fluid dynamics and original microvascular models. IVI-derived-FFR with high accuracy (88% to 94%) with strong correlations between IVI-derived-FFR and wire-based FFR (0.69 to 0.89). It may play a unique role at PCI guidance and optimization, potentially allowing comprehensive and time/cost-saving assessment of both anatomical and physiological lesion properties using a single diagnostic device.

INTRACORONARY IMAGING AND ITS USE IN INTERVENTIONAL CARDIOLOGY

SERIES OF RELATED INTEREST

Cardiology Clinics
Cardiac Electrophysiology Clinics
Heart Failure Clinics

THE CLINICS ARE NOW AVAILABLE ONLINE!
Access your subscription at:
www.theclinics.com

FOREWORD

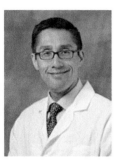

Marvin H. Eng, MD
Consulting Editor

We are pleased to introduce this issue of *Interventional Cardiology Clinics* reviewing the use of intracoronary imaging in the diagnosis, characterization, and treatment of coronary artery disease. While much progress has been made in the advancements of devices for treatment of coronary disease (eg, stents, wires), the decision-making process of coronary intervention is best driven with more detailed information gained from intracoronary imaging. While intracoronary imaging has been in use for decades, continued refinement in its utilization and growing penetration in the interventional community has made reviews such as this issue a necessity in catheterization labs.

Detailed characterization of intracoronary anatomy and plaque is now considered indispensable for percutaneous coronary interventions. Ironically, just 15 years ago, it was considered a curiosity by some, and justification for the cost of using intravascular ultrasound (IVUS) was debated. In this comprehensive issue, the practical and burgeoning applications of intracoronary imaging are explored in detail. IVUS, optical coherence tomography, and near-infrared spectroscopy are described for pragmatic clinical application as well as for continued investigation. Complete evidence basis for all three modalities are summarized for readers, and this issue can serve as the cornerstone of intracoronary imaging education for any contemporary training program.

This issue of *Interventional Cardiology Clinics* has been edited by Dr. Yasuhiro Honda, an international expert in intravascular imaging. We congratulate him on assembling an intravascular imaging compendium of the highest caliber that will no doubt set the standard for learning and teaching imaging for years to come.

Marvin H. Eng, MD
Banner University Medical Center
1111 East McDowell Road
Phoenix, AZ 85006, USA

E-mail address:
marvin.eng@bannerhealth.com

Intervent Cardiol Clin 12 (2023) xiii
https://doi.org/10.1016/j.iccl.2023.02.004
2211-7458/23/© 2023 Published by Elsevier Inc.

PREFACE

Intracoronary Imaging and Its Use in Interventional Cardiology

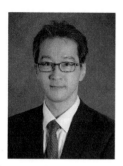

Yasuhiro Honda, MD, FACC, FAHA
Editor

In 1971, Bom and colleagues developed one of the first catheter-based real-time imaging techniques for use in the cardiac system. By placing a set of phased-array ultrasound transducers within the cardiac chambers, it was shown that higher frequencies could be used to produce high-resolution images of cardiac structures without interference from bony structures that occurs with conventional transthoracic ultrasound imaging. By the late 1980s, my mentor at Stanford, Prof Paul G. Yock, and his colleagues had successfully miniaturized a single-transducer intravascular ultrasound (IVUS) catheter system to enable the transducer placement within coronary arteries. Over the decades since then, IVUS has become a pivotal catheter-based imaging technology worldwide, having provided practical guidance for percutaneous interventions as well as scientific insights into vascular biology in clinical settings. During this period, several other advanced imaging technologies were also developed and introduced into the clinical arena, including catheter-based optical coherence tomography (OCT), an optical analog of IVUS offering greater axial resolution at the expense of beam penetration, and intravascular near-infrared spectroscopy (NIRS), which is specifically designed to identify the lipid component within the vessel wall. While current evidence regarding the impact of intracoronary imaging on cardiovascular outcomes is founded mostly on the results of clinical IVUS studies due to its longest history in clinical application, solid data are rapidly accumulating to support the benefits of the newer imaging technologies as well.

This issue of *Interventional Cardiology Clinics* is therefore intended to serve as an up-to-date resource of IVUS, OCT, and NIRS, not only for practicing cardiologists, residents, and students but also for researchers and engineers with aspirations to apply or advance these sophisticated catheter-based imaging technologies. In each modality, experts in the field discuss its diagnostic application, specifically focusing on vulnerable plaque and acute coronary syndrome, its practical application, and latest evidence in image-guided percutaneous coronary intervention, as well as ongoing technical efforts to further enhance the utility of the principal imaging technology. Furthermore, the use of intravascular imaging in other specific applications is addressed in dedicated articles, such as cardiac allograft vasculopathy, symptomatic myocardial bridging, and imaging-derived coronary physiology assessment. Despite recent advancements in noninvasive imaging allowing rapid and detailed visualization of cardiovascular structures, clinical demand for catheter-based imaging is growing, largely driven by increasing complexity of target lesions for percutaneous interventions as well as evolving treatment technologies that require precise

Intervent Cardiol Clin 12 (2023) xv–xvi
https://doi.org/10.1016/j.iccl.2023.01.002
2211-7458/23/© 2023 Published by Elsevier Inc.

procedural guidance or real-time assessment of the treatment effects. It is my hope that this focused issue will prove useful to the medical and health care engineering community, in its effort to serve as a comprehensive guide to understanding this rapidly evolving field and its role in patient care and clinical research in interventional cardiology.

Being asked to serve as the guest editor of this issue has been a great privilege. However, the successful production has required the support and cooperation of a number of individuals. I would like to express my deep appreciation to all the authors, who generously contributed their time and expert knowledge to this issue, as well as the journal editor, Dr Marvin H. Eng, and the staff of Elsevier, in particular, Ms Arlene B. Campos and Ms Joanna Collett. Without their expertise, dedication, and time commitment, this issue would not have been possible.

Yasuhiro Honda, MD, FACC, FAHA
Cardiovascular Core Analysis Laboratory
Division of Cardiovascular Medicine
Stanford Cardiovascular Institute
Stanford University School of Medicine
300 Pasteur Drive, Room H3554
Stanford, CA 94305, USA

E-mail address:
yshonda@stanford.edu

Intravascular Ultrasound in Vulnerable Plaque and Acute Coronary Syndrome

Kozo Okada, MD, PhD, Kiyoshi Hibi, MD, PhD*

KEYWORDS

• Acute coronary syndromes • Vulnerable plaque • Plaque disruption • IVUS • RF-IVUS

KEY POINTS

• Vulnerable plaque plays a crucial role in the development of acute coronary syndrome (ACS).
• The detection of vulnerable plaque is quite important to better understand the pathogenesis of ACS and to further improve ACS management.
• Intravascular ultrasound (IVUS) is a well-established device to identify vulnerable plaque and to understand the pathophysiology of ACS.
• IVUS has been used to establish risk factors associated with vulnerable plaque and future cardiac events, and to evaluate the efficacy of pharmacologic interventions for stabilizing vulnerable plaque.

INTRODUCTION

Despite recent advances in percutaneous coronary intervention (PCI) and medical treatments, acute coronary syndrome (ACS) remains a leading cause of mortality and morbidity worldwide and continues to be a substantial proportion of the global disease burden.[1] Although ACS refers to a large spectrum of clinical conditions, including unstable angina, acute myocardial infarction (AMI), and sudden cardiac death, its comprehensive disease concept is primarily characterized by acute myocardial ischemia caused by plaque disruption and consequent thrombosis-induced severe coronary artery stenosis or occlusion.[1] Vulnerable plaque is widely accepted to be susceptible to plaque disruption and thrombosis and to play a pivotal role in the pathogenesis of ACS, being responsible for most ACS.[1,2] These concepts have evolved with the results of advancements in basic and clinical investigations along with the development and rapid expansion of invasive as well as noninvasive coronary imaging modalities, seeking the ability to detect high-risk plaques

(ie, vulnerable plaques) before their disruption and formation of an occlusive thrombus.[2] Although coronary angiography (CAG) is widely used to evaluate the degrees of coronary artery disease (CAD), it provides only indirect information on vessel wall structures and is unable to identify the detailed features of vulnerable plaques. Retrospective studies of patients presenting with AMI underscore this limitation by reporting that AMI frequently develops in previously nonsevere stenotic lesions.[3] In contrast, intracoronary imaging can potentially distinguish vulnerable plaques from benign types of plaques. Given its superior resolution compared with noninvasive imaging, intracoronary imaging modalities, such as intravascular ultrasound (IVUS), optical coherence tomography (OCT), near-infrared spectroscopy (NIRS), and intracoronary endoscopy, have been used to evaluate culprit lesions of ACS (Table 1).[2] Among them, IVUS has been the first widely applied clinical technology with sufficient tissue penetration to directly visualize the entire coronary vessel-wall structures.[4] IVUS has also enabled area and volume measurements (vessel, plaque, and

---

Division of Cardiology, Yokohama City University Medical Center
* Corresponding author. 4-57 Urafune-cho, Minami-ku, Yokohama 232-0024, Japan.
E-mail address: hibikiyo@yokohama-cu.ac.jp

Intervent Cardiol Clin 12 (2023) 155–165
https://doi.org/10.1016/j.iccl.2022.10.003
2211-7458/23/

Table 1
Comparison of intravascular imaging modalities for detection of vulnerable plaque features

Vulnerable Plaque Features	Grayscale IVUS	RF-IVUS	NIRS-IVUS	OCT	Angioscopy
Plaque disruption	++	++	++	+++	++
Thrombus	++	++	++	+++	++
Lipid-rich necrotic core	+	++	+++	++	++
Thin-fibrous cap	-	-/+	-	+++	++
Inflammation (macrophage)	-	-	-	++	-
Cholesterol cleft	-	-	-	++	-
Positive remodeling	+++	+++	+++	+	-
Plaque burden	+++	+++	+++	+	-
Spotty calcification	++	++	++	+	-
Intraplaque hemorrhage	+	+	+	+	-
Neovascularization	-	-	-	+	-

Indicator – means "not distinguishable"; + means "barely distinguishable"; ++ means "moderately distinguishable"; +++ means "well delineated".
Abbreviation: NIRS-IVUS, near-infrared spectroscopy intravascular ultrasound.

lumen areas and volumes) of region of interest because it has an intrinsic distance calibration. These advantages of IVUS enable us to interrogate biological processes, such as plaque burden, plaque eccentricity, plaque composition, vessel remodeling, and the mechanisms of thrombosis (ie, plaque rupture, plaque erosion, and calcified nodule), as well as plaque progression and regression, contributing to the growing evidence on the process of atherosclerosis. This article reviews current clinical evidence established by IVUS and the recent advancements in our understanding of vulnerable plaque and its role in ACS management.

HISTOPATHOLOGICAL FEATURES OF VULNERABLE PLAQUE

Since the early pioneering study uncovering the pivotal role of plaque rupture and coronary thrombosis as the major cause of ACS and sudden cardiac death, the concept of vulnerable plaque has evolved with the continuous update of relevant terminology.[5] As mentioned earlier, lesions that eventually cause a coronary occlusion in the setting of ACS are often unsuspicious on previous CAG, frequently demonstrating low-grade stenoses,[3] and in 1989, James E. Muller and colleagues termed for the first time these hemodynamically insignificant plaques as vulnerable plaques.[6] Previous histopathological studies have also identified 3 distinct causes of luminal thrombosis, namely plaque rupture, erosion, and calcified nodules.[5,7,8] Although plaque rupture is the principal mechanism that accounts for ACS,[8] the term "vulnerable plaque" is described broadly enough to include all dangerous plaques at risk for thrombosis or rapid progression to become culprit lesions,[9] which has been widely adopted by investigators and clinicians.

Various histopathological features of vulnerable plaques are comprehensively summarized in a previous consensus document in 2003.[9] Morphologic features of vulnerable plaques have been identified as a large lipid/necrotic core with a thin fibrous cap (<65 μm), known as thin cap fibroatheroma (TCFA), large lipid contents, the presence of active inflammation (infiltration of macrophages and lymphocytes within the plaque, and the degradation of the endothelium), positive remodeling, intraplaque hemorrhage, cholesterol crystals/clefts, microcalcification, and neovascularization, although the histopathological description of vulnerable plaque lacks definitive proof of prospective physiologic data confirming a cause-and-effect relationship.[5,8–10] Lesions with significant stenosis ($>90\%$ diameter stenosis) are also considered vulnerable plaques because rapid progression could lead to clinical events.[9] Among these morphologic features, TCFA is a critical hallmark of vulnerable plaque, which is most likely to rupture and accounts for 60% to 70% of acute coronary thrombosis events.[5,8]

DETECTION OF VULNERABLE PLAQUE BY INTRAVASCULAR ULTRASOUND
Plaque Phenotypes
Based on echogenicity, coronary plaques are classified into soft, fibrous, calcified, and mixed

plaques by grayscale IVUS (Fig. 1).[11] Advanced tissue characterization techniques on computer-assisted radiofrequency (RF) signal analysis can provide a more accurate detection of vulnerable plaque components and appreciation of the long-term impact of plaque composition on clinical outcomes.[11] Virtual Histology™ (VH) IVUS system (Philips Volcano Corp., USA) classifies plaques as 4 types: fibrous, necrotic, calcific, and fibrofatty; Integrated Backscatter (IB) IVUS (Terumo Corp., Japan) uses integrated backscatter values to differentiate 4 tissue types: calcification, fibrosis, dense fibrosis, and lipid pool; and iMap™ system (Boston Scientific Corp., USA) identifies and quantifies 4 different types of atherosclerotic components (fibrotic, necrotic, lipidic, and calcified tissues), although iMAP system is commercially unavailable (Fig. 2). Additionally, NIRS is specifically designed for the detection of lipid-rich plaque (LRP; also known as lipid core plaque [LCP]), which is visualized as a summary of the probability displayed in a 2-dimensional color map of the vessel called a "chemogram" with the spatial (circumferential and longitudinal) information (see Fig. 2).[11] All these systems have demonstrated a correlation between imaging-derived plaque compositions and corresponding histopathology of coronary specimens.[11]

Thin Cap Fibroatheroma

Histologically, TCFA is characterized by the combination of a thin fibrous cap and a large lipid or necrotic core containing numerous cholesterol clefts.[9] Although the exact cap thickness cannot be measured with IVUS due to the limited axial resolution, an alternative definition for TCFA has been proposed by VH-IVUS, which comprised plaques with a plaque burden of greater than 40% and a large necrotic-rich core (>10%), without apparent overlying fibrotic tissue seen on at least 3 consecutive frames.[12–14] Previous clinical studies have demonstrated that VH-IVUS-determined TCFAs are more frequently seen in patients with ACS than those with stable CAD and more often found in the proximal segments of coronary arteries.[12] The Providing Regional Observations to Study Predictors of Events in the Coronary Tree (PROSPECT) trial, the first large-scale prospective trial to provide a natural history study of vulnerable plaque, used 3-vessel IVUS imaging in 700 patients with ACS and identified 3 baseline IVUS characteristics that independently predicted events: (1) plaque burden greater than 70% (hazard ratio [HR] = 5.03), (2) VH-determined TCFA (HR = 3.35), and (3) minimal luminal area less

than 4.0 mm^2 (HR = 3.21).[13] Major adverse cardiovascular events (MACE) also occurred in 18% of lesions that had all 3 of these characteristics and in less than 1% of lesions with none of them. Several other prospective studies confirmed the results by demonstrating that VH-determined TCFA was again associated with an increased occurrence of cardiac events.[14]

Lipid Accumulation

Multiple clinical studies have shown that increased lipid volumes are related to unstable lesion characteristics, clinical presentations, and future adverse events. A previous study of IB-IVUS found greater percent lipid and smaller percent fibrous volumes, in addition to increased plaque eccentricity, plaque burden, and remodeling index, in lesions in patients with ACS versus stable angina pectoris (SAP).[15,16] Higher lipid contents of coronary plaques by IB-IVUS have been also associated with ACS and an increased risk of sustaining nonculprit-lesion (NCL)-related ischemic events and MACE.[17,18] Larger lipidic and necrotic components with a smaller fibrous component by iMAP analysis were seen in the culprit lesions in patients with versus without ACS.[19] Another investigation of 95 patients who underwent PCI reported that increased necrotic plaque volume by iMAP analysis was an independent predictor of slow-flow during PCI and that the cutoff value of necrotic plaque volume for predicting slow-flow was 21.6 mm^3 (sensitivity of 81.8% and specificity of 61.9%).[20] LRP (or LCP) by NIRS has been frequently observed in patients with ACS versus SAP as well.[21] Most culprit lesions of ST-segment elevation myocardial infarction (STEMI) are also characterized by a large, often circumferential, LRP concentrated at the culprit site and a maximum lipid core burden index (LCBI) over a 4 mm length (maxLCBI$_{4mm}$) of greater than 400 was found to be a signature of plaques causing STEMI.[22] A large, prospective, multicenter study of 898 patients with recent myocardial infarction (PROSPECT-II) identified lesions with a high lipid content and large plaque burden as lesions at the highest risk for NLC-related MACE.[23]

Attenuated-Signal Plaque and Echolucent Plaque

Attenuated-signal plaque (ASP) is defined as a hypoechoic plaque with noncalcium-related, ultrasound signal attenuation (see Fig. 1).[24] ASP likely represents the presence of necrotic core, lipid pool, and advanced atherosclerosis consisting predominantly of cholesterol clefts, macrophage

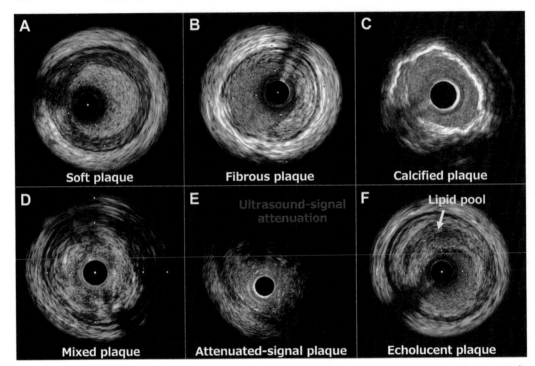

Fig. 1. Plaque phenotypes. Coronary plaques are classified into (A) soft (echogenicity less than the surrounding adventitia), (B) fibrous (intermediate echogenicity between soft plaques and calcified plaques), (C) calcified (echogenicity higher than the adventitia with acoustic shadowing), and (D) mixed plaques (more than one subtype contained within the plaque) by grayscale IVUS. (E) Attenuated-signal plaque (hypoechoic plaque with noncalcium-related, ultrasound signal attenuation). (F) Echolucent plaque (lesion containing an intraplaque low-echoic region as represented as lipid pool).

infiltration, and microcalcification.[24,25] ASP is frequently observed in ACS lesions[11] and an extended ASP is recognized as one feature of unstable atherosclerotic lesions, associated with a high rate of transient deterioration in coronary flow (ie, "slow-flow" or "no-reflow" phenomenon) by distal embolism during primary PCI, large infarct size and microvascular obstruction.[26,27] A recent prospective multicenter randomized trial (VAMPIRE 3 [Vacuum Aspiration Thrombus Removal 3]) demonstrated that distal filter protection significantly decreased the incidence of no-reflow and in-hospital serious adverse cardiac events when selectively used in patients with an ASP 5 mm or greater in length on pre-PCI IVUS.[28] Although the predictive value of baseline ASP for future cardiovascular events remains highly debatable,[29] ASP progression detected by serial IVUS imaging could be a more reliable surrogate marker for long-term prognosis. Shishikura and colleagues reported that the progression of ASP for 18 to 24 months was associated with a higher prevalence of subsequent cardiovascular events.[30] Okada, and colleagues also demonstrated, in a heart transplant study, that

patients with ASP progression during the first year after heart transplantation showed a higher incidence of acute cellular rejection within 1-year and a lower survival rate after 1-year posttransplant, compared with those without.[31]

Plaque Rupture

An occlusive thrombus formation is the final pathologic finding in most cases of ACS.[5,8] This event is usually qualified as plaque rupture, accounting for 60% to 70% of coronary thrombosis[7,8] but further causes comprise plaque erosion and calcified nodules. Plaque rupture is diagnosed when a hypoechoic cavity within the plaque is connected with the lumen and a remnant of the ruptured fibrous cap is observed at the connecting site (Fig. 3).[32] Ruptured plaques are often eccentric, less calcified, large in plaque burden, positively remodeled, and associated with large thrombi.[5,9] Previous studies have shown that multiple plaque ruptures are frequently detected by 3-vessel IVUS imaging in patients with ACS, suggesting that ACS is associated with pan-coronary destabilization.[33] Among patients with ACS, plaque rupture is

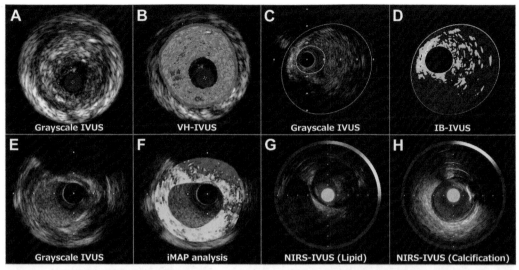

Fig. 2. Advanced plaque tissue characterization. (*A, B*) VH-IVUS classifies plaques into 4 types: fibrotic (*green*), necrotic (*red*), calcific (*white*), and fibrofatty (*yellow-green*). (*C, D*) IB-IVUS (Integrated Backscatter intravascular ultrasound) differentiates 4 tissue types: calcification (*red*), fibrosis (*green*), dense fibrosis (*yellow*), and lipid (*blue*). (*E, F*) iMap system quantifies 4 different components: fibrotic (*green*), necrotic (*pink*), lipidic (*yellow*), and calcified (*blue*). (*G, H*) NIRS-IVUS (near-infrared spectroscopy intravascular ultrasound). NIRS visualizes a summary of the probability displayed in a 2-dimensional color map of the vessel called a "chemogram" with the spatial (circumferential and longitudinal) information. A color scale from red to yellow indicates increasing algorithmic probability of the presence of lipid ranging from 0 to 1.0 for each pixel occupying 0.1 mm and 1° of the vessel wall.

more frequent and more in the proximal shoulder site in patients with STEMI compared with non-ST elevation ACS.[34] In patients with STEMI, ruptured plaques have been reported to be an independent determinant of a high incidence of no-reflow phenomenon and large infarct size.[32,35] A recent clinical study of OCT found a higher incidence of MACE in patients with plaque rupture than those with intact fibrous cap (odds ratio 3.735, confidence interval 1.358–9.735).[36]

Plaque Erosion

Plaque erosion accounts for 30% to 40% of the underlying pathologic condition of coronary thrombosis and pathologically differs from plaque rupture because it can arise without the contribution of a lesion's lipid core.[7,8] In general, plaque erosion is characterized by an eccentric plaque, which is rich in smooth muscle cells and proteoglycan, has a small necrotic/lipid core with a thick fibrous cap, usually lacks prominent inflammatory infiltrates, and less occlusive lesions.[37] These features were confirmed in clinical studies of intravascular imaging[38,39] and an OCT definition of plaque erosion was previously proposed as a plaque with an intact fibrous cap showing thrombi that allow visualization of underlying plaque.[39] A combined OCT and IVUS imaging study of

112 culprit lesions of STEMI identified that plaque erosion was seen in 30 (26.8%) lesions and was frequently associated with eccentric plaque and smaller residual thrombus after thrombolysis, and less frequently with positive remodeling.[38]

Calcified Nodule

Calcified nodule is another plaque phenotype associated with ACS, accounting for 3% to 5% of coronary thrombosis.[7,8] Calcified nodule is histologically defined as a fibrocalcific plaque with little or no underlying necrotic core, a luminal surface that is disrupted by nodules of dense calcium, and an overlying thrombus. These features have been validated on grayscale IVUS as a distinct calcification with an irregular, protruding, and convex luminal surface (see Fig. 3).[40] A subanalysis of the PROSPECT study revealed that calcified nodules were most frequently observed in midright coronary artery followed by proximal to midleft anterior descending artery, and the presence of calcified nodules was associated with the angle of bending motion of coronary artery during cardiac cycle.[41] Although its nature is yet to be fully elucidated due to the limited frequency, this study also reported that calcified nodules were less likely to develop MACE.[41]

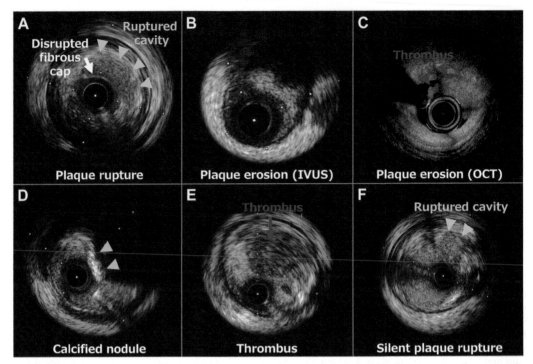

Fig. 3. Plaque rupture, erosion, and calcified nodule. (*A*) Plaque rupture. (*B*) and (*C*) Plaque erosion (corresponding IVUS and OCT images). (*D*) Calcified nodule (blue triangles). (*E*) Thrombus. (*F*) Silent plaque rupture.

Positive Remodeling

Positive remodeling, defined as the outward, abluminal expansion of the arterial wall, is a common feature of vulnerable plaque.[7] Culprit lesions responsible for ACS typically represent extensive positive remodeling, with the highest remodeling index in lesions with plaque rupture, followed by lesions with hemorrhage > TCFAs > healed plaque ruptures > fibroatheromas.[42] Multiple clinical studies have shown that preinterventional positive remodeling as assessed by IVUS predicts unfavorable acute-term and long-term outcomes after PCI.[43] A recent clinical study of combined IVUS and OCT imaging also reported a close link between positive remodeling and thinning of the fibrous cap in serial coronary examinations.[44]

Plaque Burden

Atherosclerosis is a continuous process of plaque disruption and healing. A meta-analysis of clinical and pathologic studies identified subclinical plaque rupture was detected in NCLs in 11.5% of patients with stable CAD or healthy controls, as well as 21.5% of patients with ACS.[45] Silent plaque ruptures are one of the critical triggers of phasic rather than linear progression of luminal narrowing in coronary arteries,

which may involve subclinical thrombus formation and healing.[37] These silent thrombotic events likely resulted in plaque volume progression by intramural thrombus organization rather than life-threatening ACS events. Cumulative healed plaque ruptures at the same location are clearly related to increased percent stenosis.[46] Increased plaque burden has been reported to be incrementally predictive of plaque progression, myocardial infarction, coronary revascularization, or MACE in previous clinical studies.[13,47,48]

Intraplaque Hemorrhage

Intraplaque hemorrhage may involve the critical transition from TCFA to rupture. Repeated intraplaque hemorrhage is reported to be a contributing factor to necrotic core expansion, mainly considering that red blood cell membranes serve as a potent source of free cholesterol, which is higher in disrupted plaques.[5,49] The source of hemorrhage is likely leaky vasa vasorum that infiltrates the plaque from the adventitia in response to a hypoxic environment created by increased lesion burden and inflammatory macrophages.[5] This, together with the death of macrophages, is thought to contribute to the progression of necrotic cores. High-definition IVUS may identify intraplaque hemorrhage, which seems as an echolucent area with well-delineated borders, that have a crescent shape circumscribed within the plaque.[50]

DIAGNOSTIC AND THERAPEUTIC IMPLICATIONS

One potential application of intravascular imaging could be to identify the risk factors associated with plaque progression and vulnerability related to subsequent cardiovascular outcomes as well as to evaluate novel pharmacologic interventions targeted to plaque regression and stabilization. Changes in plaque volumes and compositions measured by serial IVUS imaging have been widely used as a surrogate endpoint in clinical trials of the natural history of native coronary atherosclerosis and transplant vasculopathy and in monitoring the results of pharmacologic interventions.[2,10,47,48]

Low-density lipoprotein cholesterol (LDL-C) is a well-established risk factor for plaque vulnerability and the most important therapeutic target.[1] Multiple studies using serial IVUS imaging have revealed that the reduction of LDL-C with a statin can slow plaque progression and even promote plaque regression in a dose–response manner.[47,51,52] Clinical trials using IB-IVUS or VH-IVUS have identified that plaque stabilization by statin treatments occurs despite the lack of change in total plaque volume.[53] Other studies have suggested the anti-inflammatory effects of statin on plaque instability.[54] Multiple studies of OCT have also shown that statin therapy can thicken and harden (by calcification) the fibrous cap of LRPs.[55,56] More recently, intensive lipid-lowering treatments with a combination of statin and ezetimibe or protein convertase subtilisin kexin type 9 (PCSK9) have resulted in further plaque regression and stabilization, although controversial.[57–61]

Diabetes mellitus (DM) is also an important determinant for unfavorable clinical outcomes,[62] and plaque regression induced by statin treatment can be attenuated in patients with DM,[48] which is recognized as "residual risk." Indeed, despite achieving very low LDL-C levels ($\leq$70 mg/dL), patients with CAD were more likely to demonstrate plaque progression and have clinical events if they had DM.[48] Although DM is primarily characterized by persistent hyperglycemia, it also includes various pathologic conditions, such as insulin resistance, hyperinsulinemia, low plasma glucose-like peptide-1 levels, glucose variability, hypoglycemia, all of which have been reported to be associated with increased lipid contents and decreased

fibrous contents of coronary plaques in patients with ACS.[63–65] It was also reported that patients with DM with 3 or more major risk factors are at very high risk for cardiovascular events.[66] Therefore, an intensified multifactorial intervention of concomitant risk factors, including DM-related pathologic conditions as mentioned above, would exert favorable effects in patients with DM in terms of the degree of plaque regression.[62,67]

Metabolic syndrome with associated abdominal adiposity is also an important residual risk. Amano and colleagues reported that metabolic syndrome is associated with LRP as assessed by IB-IVUS.[68] Our group used IB-IVUS in 60 patients with ACS and identified that abnormal abdominal fat distribution (high visceral-to-subcutaneous fat ratio) was significantly correlated with increased percent lipid volumes ($r = 0.34$, $P = .008$), decreased percent fibrous volume ($r = -0.34$, $P = .007$), and thinner fibrous cap thickness ($r = -0.53$, $P \leq .0001$) by IB-IVUS.[69]

Myocardial bridging (MB) may have an interesting contribution to the development of ACS. MB is a common congenital coronary anomaly, located most frequently in the left anterior descending artery and only IVUS can precisely detect MB, both by functional assessment (systolic arterial compression) as well as a characteristic echolucent band (halo) appearance partially surrounding the artery.[70] Although most patients are presumed asymptomatic, MB can cause typical or atypical angina, arrhythmia, or ACS, most likely because of direct compressive effects on the MB segment or accelerated atherosclerosis in the segment proximal to the MB.[70–72] Our group reported the case of ACS caused by accelerated plaque formation related to MB in a young patient without apparent coronary risk factors.[72]

LIMITATIONS AND FUTURE PERSPECTIVES

IVUS has matured to become a common clinical device in current cardiac catheterization laboratories. This diagnostic modality is considerably promoting our knowledge of coronary plaque morphology, which can facilitate the rational choice of pharmacologic and local treatments as well as the endpoint assessment in specific lesions. However, there remain some limitations in its routine use in clinical practice; for example, because the current approach of imaging-based vulnerable plaque detection is primarily based on rupture-prone lesions (ie, TCFA), the precursor lesions of plaque erosion and calcified nodule (more than 30% of the cause of ACS) have not been determined yet, which possibly warrants different imaging definitions or modalities. Plaque morphology is also only one aspect that determines a plaque's fate, and multiple other factors and conditions related to the occurrence of ACS, such as coronary flow dynamics, intrinsic hemostatic/fibrinolytic dysfunction, neurohormonal dysregulation, and environmental factors and triggers, can contribute to subsequent thrombus enlargement and final luminal occlusion.[2] Therefore, it is unlikely that plaque vulnerability alone can reliably predict the outcome for a specific plaque.[73] It is also challenging to determine at an early stage if atherosclerotic plaque will become unstable and vulnerable.[10] In contrast, multimodality hybrid imaging modalities may overcome these inherent limitations. The combined imaging system of IVUS and NIRS, as well as IVUS and OCT catheters, is an example enabling the analysis of both vessel structure and plaque composition simultaneously. Both anatomic and functional assessments of CAD by intravascular imaging with the function of artificial intelligence (AI)-assisted auto lumen detection may represent alternative future directions. For example, the feasibility of RF-IVUS analysis of blood signals to estimate functional ischemia of intermediate stenoses has been previously reported.[74] The support of machine learning with AI could also be useful to combine the intravascular imaging findings and biomarkers (genetic or plasma proteins) and identify the factors associated with plaque vulnerability/progression and future ACS onset. Although some of these emerging technologies are yet to mature, the advances in diagnostic modalities will enable us to comprehensively understand the pathophysiology of ACS and further enhance a framework for better triage, future tailoring of medications, and more efficient, personalized therapy for our patients.

SUMMARY

Again, the detection of vulnerable plaque is quite important to better understand the pathogenesis of ACS and to further improve ACS management. To implement the intravascular imaging modalities as a screening tool to guide primary or secondary prevention therapies, future studies should focus on optimizing imaging techniques and evaluating the effectiveness of vulnerable plaque stabilization on clinical endpoints; in other words, whether vulnerable plaque features are modifiable and plaque rupture can be prevented.

CLINICS CARE POINTS

- IVUS enables us to interrogate biological processes, such as plaque burden, plaque eccentricity, plaque composition, vessel remodeling, and the mechanisms of thrombosis (i.e., plaque rupture, plaque erosion, and calcified nodule), as well as plaque progression and regression.

- Changes in plaque volumes and compositions measured by serial IVUS imaging have been widely used as a surrogate endpoint in clinical trials of the natural history of native coronary atherosclerosis and transplant vasculopathy and in monitoring the results of pharmacological interventions.

- IVUS may enhance the identification of high-risk patients susceptible to future cardiac events.

DISCLOSURE

No conflict of interest with regard to this article.

REFERENCES

1. Kimura K, Kimura T, Ishihara M, et al. JCS 2018 guideline on diagnosis and treatment of acute coronary syndrome. Circ J 2019;83(5):1085–196. Published online.
2. Sakamoto A, Cornelissen A, Sato Y, et al. Vulnerable plaque in patients with acute coronary syndrome: identification, importance, and management. Us Cardiol Rev 2022;16. https://doi.org/10.15420/usc.2021.22.
3. Ambrose JA, Tannenbaum MA, Alexopoulos D, et al. Angiographic progression of coronary artery disease and the development of myocardial infarction. J Am Coll Cardiol 1988;12(1):56–62.
4. Sonoda S, Hibi K, Okura H, et al. Current clinical use of intravascular ultrasound imaging to guide percutaneous coronary interventions. Cardiovasc intervention Ther 2019;35(1):30–6. Published online.
5. Finn AV, Nakano M, Narula J, et al. Concept of vulnerable/unstable plaque. Arterioscler Thromb Vasc Biol 2010;30(7):1282–92.
6. Muller JE, Tofler GH, Stone PH. Circadian variation and triggers of onset of acute cardiovascular disease. Circulation 1989;79(4):733–43.
7. Virmani R, Burke AP, Farb A, et al. Pathology of the vulnerable plaque. J Am Coll Cardiol 2006;47(8 Suppl):C13–8.
8. Virmani R, Kolodgie FD, Burke AP, et al. Lessons from sudden coronary death: a comprehensive

morphological classification scheme for atherosclerotic lesions. Arterioscler Thromb Vasc Biol 2000; 20(5):1262–75.

9. Naghavi M, Libby P, Falk E, et al. From Vulnerable Plaque to Vulnerable Patient A Call for New Definitions and Risk Assessment Strategies: Part I. Circulation 2003;108(14):1664–72.

10. Hafiane A. Vulnerable plaque, characteristics, detection, and potential therapies. J Cardiovasc Dev Dis 2019;6(3). https://doi.org/10.3390/jcdd6030026.

11. Honda S, Kataoka Y, Kanaya T, et al. Characterization of coronary atherosclerosis by intravascular imaging modalities. Cardiovasc Diagn Ther 2016;6(4): 368–81.

12. Rodriguez-Granillo GA, García-García HM, Fadden EPM, et al. In Vivo intravascular ultrasound-derived thin-cap fibroatheroma detection using ultrasound radiofrequency data analysis. J Am Coll Cardiol 2005;46(11):2038–42.

13. Stone GW, Maehara A, Lansky AJ, et al. A prospective natural-history study of coronary atherosclerosis. N Engl J Med 2011;364(3):226–35.

14. Calvert PA, Obaid DR, O'Sullivan M, et al. Association between IVUS findings and adverse outcomes in patients with coronary artery disease: the VIVA (VH-IVUS in Vulnerable Atherosclerosis) Study. JACC Cardiovasc Imaging 2011;4(8):894–901.

15. Sano K, Kawasaki M, Ishihara Y, et al. Assessment of vulnerable plaques causing acute coronary syndrome using integrated backscatter intravascular ultrasound. J Am Coll Cardiol 2006;47(4):734–41.

16. Maejima N, Hibi K, Saka K, et al. Morphological features of non-culprit plaques on optical coherence tomography and integrated backscatter intravascular ultrasound in patients with acute coronary syndromes. Eur Hear J Cardiovasc Imaging 2015; 16(2):190–7.

17. Amano T, Matsubara T, Uetani T, et al. Lipid-rich plaques predict non-target-lesion ischemic events in patients undergoing percutaneous coronary intervention. Circ J 2011;75(1):157–66.

18. Tashiro H, Tanaka A, Ishii H, et al. Lipid-rich large plaques in a non-culprit left main coronary artery and long-term clinical outcomes. Int J Cardiol 2020;305:5–10.

19. Kozuki A, Shinke T, Otake H, et al. Feasibility of a novel radiofrequency signal analysis for in-vivo plaque characterization in humans: Comparison of plaque components between patients with and without acute coronary syndrome. Int J Cardiol 2013;167(4):1591–6.

20. Utsunomiya M, Hara H, Sugi K, et al. Relationship between tissue characterisations with 40 MHz intravascular ultrasound imaging and slow flow during coronary intervention. Eurointervention 2011;7(3):340–6.

21. Madder RD, Smith JL, Dixon SR, et al. Composition of target lesions by near-infrared spectroscopy in patients with acute coronary syndrome versus stable angina. Circ Cardiovasc Interv 2012;5(1):55–61.

22. Madder RD, Goldstein JA, Madden SP, et al. Detection by near-infrared spectroscopy of large lipid core plaques at culprit sites in patients with acute ST-segment elevation myocardial infarction. JACC Cardiovasc interventions 2013;6(8):838–46.

23. Erlinge D, Maehara A, Ben-Yehuda O, et al. Identification of vulnerable plaques and patients by intracoronary near-infrared spectroscopy and ultrasound (PROSPECT II): a prospective natural history study. Lancet 2021;397(10278):985–95.

24. Honda Y. Intravascular imaging to guide PCI for acute myocardial infarction shifting from "whether" to "how". Jacc Cardiovasc Interventions 2021; 14(22):2444–6.

25. Pu J, Mintz GS, Biro S, et al. Insights into echo-attenuated plaques, echolucent plaques, and plaques with spotty calcification: novel findings from comparisons among intravascular ultrasound, near-infrared spectroscopy, and pathological histology in 2,294 human coronary artery segments. J Am Coll Cardiol 2014;63(21):2220–33.

26. Endo M, Hibi K, Shimizu T, et al. Impact of ultrasound attenuation and plaque rupture as detected by intravascular ultrasound on the incidence of no-reflow phenomenon after percutaneous coronary intervention in ST-segment elevation myocardial infarction. JACC Cardiovasc interventions 2010; 3(5):540–9.

27. Shiono Y, Kubo T, Tanaka A, et al. Impact of attenuated plaque as detected by intravascular ultrasound on the occurrence of microvascular obstruction after percutaneous coronary intervention in patients with st-segment elevation myocardial infarction. Jacc Cardiovasc Interventions 2013; 6(8):847–53.

28. Hibi K, Kozuma K, Sonoda S, et al. A randomized study of distal filter protection versus conventional treatment during percutaneous coronary intervention in patients with attenuated plaque identified by intravascular ultrasound. JACC Cardiovasc interventions 2018;11(16):1545–55.

29. Xu K, Mintz GS, Kubo T, et al. Long-term follow-up of attenuated plaques in patients with acute myocardial infarction: an intravascular ultrasound substudy of the HORIZONS-AMI trial. Circ Cardiovasc Interv 2012;5(2):185–92.

30. Shishikura D, Kataoka Y, Giovanni GD, et al. Progression of ultrasound plaque attenuation and low echogenicity associates with major adverse cardiovascular events. Eur Heart J 2020;41(31):2965–73.

31. Okada K, Fearon WF, Luikart H, et al. Attenuated-Signal plaque progression predicts long-term mortality after heart transplantation ivus assessment of cardiac allograft vasculopathy. J Am Coll Cardiol 2016;68(4):382–92.

32. Kusama I, Hibi K, Kosuge M, et al. Impact of plaque rupture on infarct size in ST-segment elevation anterior acute myocardial infarction. J Am Coll Cardiol 2007;50(13):1230–7.

33. Rioufol G, Finet G, Ginon I, et al. Multiple atherosclerotic plaque rupture in acute coronary syndrome: a three-vessel intravascular ultrasound study. Circulation 2002;106(7):804–8.

34. Fang C, Yin Y, Jiang S, et al. Increased Vulnerability and distinct layered phenotype at culprit and non-culprit lesions in STEMI versus NSTEMI. Jacc Cardiovasc Imaging 2022;15(4):672–81.

35. Okada K, Hibi K, Kikuchi S, et al. Culprit Lesion Morphology of Rapidly Progressive and Extensive Anterior-Wall ST-Segment Elevation Myocardial Infarction. Circ Cardiovasc Imaging 2022;15(11):e014497.

36. Niccoli G, Montone RA, Vito LD, et al. Plaque rupture and intact fibrous cap assessed by optical coherence tomography portend different outcomes in patients with acute coronary syndrome. Eur Heart J 2015;36(22):1377–84.

37. Vergallo R, Crea F. Atherosclerotic Plaque Healing. N Engl J Med 2020;383(9):846–57.

38. Higuma T, Soeda T, Abe N, et al. A combined optical coherence tomography and intravascular ultrasound study on plaque rupture, plaque erosion, and calcified nodule in patients with ST-segment elevation myocardial infarction: incidence, morphologic characteristics, and outcomes after percutaneous coronary intervention. JACC Cardiovasc interventions 2015;8(9):1166–76.

39. Kubo T, Imanishi T, Takarada S, et al. Assessment of culprit lesion morphology in acute myocardial infarction: ability of optical coherence tomography compared with intravascular ultrasound and coronary angioscopy. J Am Coll Cardiol 2007;50(10):933–9.

40. Lee JB, Mintz GS, Lisauskas JB, et al. Histopathologic Validation of the intravascular ultrasound diagnosis of calcified coronary artery nodules. Am J Cardiol 2011;108(11):1547–51.

41. Xu Y, Mintz GS, Tam A, et al. Prevalence, distribution, predictors, and outcomes of patients with calcified nodules in native coronary arteries. Circulation 2012;126(5):537–45.

42. Burke AP, Kolodgie FD, Farb A, et al. Morphological predictors of arterial remodeling in coronary atherosclerosis. Circulation 2002;105(3):297–303.

43. Okura H, Morino Y, Oshima A, et al. Preintervention arterial remodeling affects clinical outcome following stenting: an intravascular ultrasound study. J Am Coll Cardiol 2001;37(4):1031–5.

44. Yamada R, Okura H, Kume T, et al. Relationship between arterial and fibrous cap remodeling: a serial three-vessel intravascular ultrasound and optical coherence tomography study. Circ Cardiovasc Interv 2010;3(5):484–90.

45. Arbab-Zadeh A, Fuster V. The myth of the "vulnerable plaque" transitioning from a focus on individual lesions to atherosclerotic disease burden for coronary artery disease risk assessment. J Am Coll Cardiol 2015;65(8):846–55.

46. Burke AP, Kolodgie FD, Farb A, et al. Healed plaque ruptures and sudden coronary death. Circulation 2001;103(7):934–40.

47. Nicholls SJ, Hsu A, Wolski K, et al. Intravascular ultrasound-derived measures of coronary atherosclerotic plaque burden and clinical outcome. J Am Coll Cardiol 2010;55(21):2399–407.

48. Bayturan O, Kapadia S, Nicholls SJ, et al. Clinical predictors of plaque progression despite very low levels of low-density lipoprotein cholesterol. J Am Coll Cardiol 2010;55(24):2736–42.

49. Kolodgie FD, Gold HK, Burke AP, et al. Intraplaque hemorrhage and progression of coronary atheroma. N Engl J Med 2003;349(24):2316–25.

50. Ohashi H, Ando H, Otsuka F, et al. Histopathologically confirmed intraplaque haemorrhage in a patient with unstable angina. Eur Hear J Cardiovasc Imaging 2022;23(4):e165.

51. Ahmadi A, Narula J. Primary and secondary prevention, or subclinical and clinical atherosclerosis. JACC Cardiovasc Imaging 2017;10(4):447–50.

52. O'Keefe JH, Cordain L, Harris WH, et al. Optimal low-density lipoprotein is 50 to 70 mg/dl: lower is better and physiologically normal. J Am Coll Cardiol 2004;43(11):2142–6.

53. Kawasaki M, Sano K, Okubo M, et al. Volumetric quantitative analysis of tissue characteristics of coronary plaques after statin therapy using three-dimensional integrated backscatter intravascular ultrasound. J Am Coll Cardiol 2005;45(12):1946–53.

54. Puri R, Nissen SE, Libby P, et al. C-Reactive protein, but not low-density lipoprotein cholesterol levels, associate with coronary atheroma regression and cardiovascular events after maximally intensive statin therapy. Circulation 2013;128(22):2395–403.

55. Komukai K, Kubo T, Kitabata H, et al. Effect of atorvastatin therapy on fibrous cap thickness in coronary atherosclerotic plaque as assessed by optical coherence tomography: the EASY-FIT study. J Am Coll Cardiol 2014;64(21):2207–17.

56. Puri R, Nicholls SJ, Shao M, et al. Impact of statins on serial coronary calcification during atheroma progression and regression. J Am Coll Cardiol 2015;65(13):1273–82.

57. Nicholls SJ, Puri R, Anderson T, et al. Effect of evolocumab on coronary plaque composition. J Am Coll Cardiol 2018;72(17):2012–21.

58. Gao F, Wang ZJ, Ma XT, et al. Effect of alirocumab on coronary plaque in patients with coronary artery disease assessed by optical coherence tomography. Lipids Health Dis 2021;20(1):106.

59. Tsujita K, Sugiyama S, Sumida H, et al. Impact of dual lipid-lowering strategy with ezetimibe and atorvastatin on coronary plaque regression in patients with percutaneous coronary intervention the multicenter randomized controlled PRECISE-IVUS trial. J Am Coll Cardiol 2015;66(5):495–507.

60. Ako J, Hibi K, Tsujita K, et al. Effect of alirocumab on coronary atheroma volume in japanese patients with acute coronary syndrome - the ODYSSEY J-IVUS trial. Circ J 2019;83(10):2025–33.

61. Hibi K, Sonoda S, Kawasaki M, et al. Effects of ezetimibe-statin combination therapy on coronary atherosclerosis in acute coronary syndrome. Circ J 2018;82(3):757–66.

62. Ueki K, Sasako T, Okazaki Y, et al. Effect of an intensified multifactorial intervention on cardiovascular outcomes and mortality in type 2 diabetes (J-DOIT3): an open-label, randomised controlled trial. Lancet Diabetes Endocrinol 2017;5(12):951–64.

63. Mitsuhashi T, Hibi K, Konishi M, et al. Plasma glucagon-like peptide-1 and tissue characteristics of coronary plaque in non-diabetic acute coronary syndrome patients. Circ J 2016;80(2):469–76.

64. Mitsuhashi T, Hibi K, Kosuge M, et al. Relation between hyperinsulinemia and nonculprit plaque characteristics in nondiabetic patients with acute coronary syndromes. JACC Cardiovasc Imaging 2011;4(4):392–401.

65. Okada K, Hibi K, Gohbara M, et al. Association between blood glucose variability and coronary plaque instability in patients with acute coronary syndromes. Cardiovasc Diabetol 2015;14(1):111.

66. Cosentino F, Grant PJ, Aboyans V, et al. 2019 ESC Guidelines on diabetes, pre-diabetes, and cardiovascular diseases developed in collaboration with the EASD. Eur Heart J 2020;41(2):255–323.

67. Okada K, Kikuchi S, Kuji S, et al. Impact of early intervention with alogliptin on coronary plaque regression and stabilization in patients with acute coronary syndromes. Atherosclerosis 2022;360:1–7.

68. Amano T, Matsubara T, Uetani T, et al. Impact of metabolic syndrome on tissue characteristics of angiographically mild to moderate coronary lesions integrated backscatter intravascular ultrasound study. J Am Coll Cardiol 2007;49(11):1149–56.

69. Okada K, Hibi K, Honda Y, et al. Association between abdominal fat distribution and coronary plaque instability in patients with acute coronary syndrome. Nutr Metab Cardiovasc Dis 2020;30(7):1169–78.

70. Yamada R, Tremmel JA, Tanaka S, et al. Functional versus anatomic assessment of myocardial bridging by intravascular ultrasound: impact of arterial compression on proximal atherosclerotic plaque. J Am Hear Assoc Cardiovasc Cerebrovasc Dis 2016;5(4):e001735.

71. Okada K, Hibi K, Ogino Y, et al. Impact of myocardial bridge on life-threatening ventricular arrhythmia in patients with implantable cardioverter defibrillator. J Am Hear Assoc Cardiovasc Cerebrovasc Dis 2020;9(21):e017455.

72. Kikuchi S, Okada K, Hibi K, et al. Myocardial infarction caused by accelerated plaque formation related to myocardial bridge in a young man. Can J Cardiol 2018;34(12):1687.e13–5.

73. Suh WM, Seto AH, Margey RJP, et al. Intravascular detection of the vulnerable plaque. Circ Cardiovasc Imaging 2011;4(2):169–78.

74. Okada K, Hibi K, Matsushita K, et al. Intravascular ultrasound radiofrequency signal analysis of blood speckles: Physiological assessment of intermediate coronary artery stenosis. Catheter Cardiovasc Interv 2020;96(2):E155–64.

Intravascular Ultrasound-Guided Percutaneous Coronary Intervention: Practical Application

Shinjo Sonoda, MD, PhD*, Koichi Node, MD, PhD

KEYWORDS

- Intravascular ultrasound • Optical coherence tomography • Percutaneous coronary intervention
- Drug-eluting stent • In-stent restenosis • Coronary angiography • Minimum stent area
- Troubleshooting

KEY POINTS

- Pre-PCI IVUS can evaluate underlying plaque characteristics to determine the necessity of lesion preparation and the risk of distal embolization that can cause periprocedural myocardial infarction, in addition to providing the morphometric information required for precise device sizing.
- Post-DES IVUS can detect findings related to stent failure, such as stent underexpansion, incomplete strut apposition, residual plaque and/or dissection at stent edge, and in-stent tissue protrusion.
- To avoid the IVUS catheter being stuck during complex PCI, operators should make sure to return the imaging core to the tip after observation, keep rotating the transducer, and slowly retrieve the catheter while checking with fluoroscopy.
- To further improve the outcome of PCI, it is important to learn how to use IVUS properly and successfully in various situations.

INTRODUCTION

Intracoronary imaging modalities, such as intravascular ultrasonography (IVUS) and optical coherence tomography (OCT), provide detailed information on coronary lesions during percutaneous coronary intervention (PCI) procedures. These modalities are commonly used for stent optimization after drug-eluting stent (DES) implantation and to determine the cause of stent thrombosis or in-stent restenosis (ISR). These imaging modalities also provide useful information for predicting possible complications and how to deal with complications when they occur. To date, multiple studies have shown that intracoronary imaging improves clinical outcomes following PCI.[1,2] In this article, the authors summarize the practical application of IVUS, including standard usage in their daily clinical practice and how to use IVUS in particular situations.

STANDARD INTRAVASCULAR ULTRASOUND USAGE

IVUS generates cross-sectional images of the coronary arteries. Coronary angiography (CAG) can obtain luminal information only, whereas IVUS provides complementary short-axis information of lumen, plaque, and vessel wall. Because of the side-looking catheter design, it must be introduced across the target segment to obtain lesion images. In coronary arteries, IVUS with mechanically rotating high-resolution (60 MHz) transducer is commonly used.

Department of Cardiovascular Medicine, Saga University, 5-1-1 Nabeshima, Saga 849-8501, Japan
* Corresponding author.
E-mail address: ssonoda@cc.saga-u.ac.jp

Intervent Cardiol Clin 12 (2023) 167–175
https://doi.org/10.1016/j.iccl.2022.12.001
2211-7458/23/© 2022 Elsevier Inc. All rights reserved.

Transducer pullback can be conducted manually or by using a motorized pullback system (faster pullbacks of 2.5–10 mm/s are available in some latest-generation systems).

The most useful feature of IVUS over OCT is its ability to visualize the entire vessel wall in most cases owing to the deeper tissue penetration of ultrasound signals. The operators need to know how to use IVUS in optimizing PCI outcomes (4 checkpoints: stent sizing, stenting site and length, good expansion, and no edge injury). In the DES era, smaller stent sizes and longer stent lengths are often selected for their delivery performance and for full lesion coverage, respectively. After DES implantation, it is crucial to determine the optimal end point in each lesion. It is recommended that IVUS be inserted far distal to the stent and that the entire vessel be scanned with slow-speed (0.5–1 mm/s) automated pullback to the ostium. If necessary, the minimum stent area (MSA) should be measured and it should be evaluated whether postdilation or additional stent placement is required (Table 1).[3]

INTRAVASCULAR ULTRASOUND-GUIDED PERCUTANEOUS CORONARY INTERVENTION

Before Stent Implantation

IVUS observation before PCI can elucidate underlying plaque characteristics to determine the necessity of lesion preparation.[4] In particular, diagnosis of calcified lesions is important and easily performed with IVUS, although the thickness of calcium is usually unmeasurable by IVUS due to acoustic shadowing behind the calcium. However, the extension of superficial calcium arc greater than or equal to 180° represents a strong indication of prestenting adjunctive calcium modification with rotational/orbital atherectomy or cutting/scoring balloons.[4,5] IVUS is also useful to predict high-risk patients for postprocedural myocardial infarction, distal embolization, or no reflow phenomenon during PCI. In particular, lipid-rich plaque with echo attenuation, also known as attenuated signal plaque (ASP), has been recognized as one of the morphologic predictors of postprocedural myocardial infarction (Fig. 1).[6,7] In patients with acute coronary syndrome (ACS) and stable coronary artery disease, the prevalence of ASP was reported as approximately 45% and 30%, respectively.[8] In a consecutive series of patients with ST-segment elevation myocardial infarction, ASP greater than or equal to 180° in arc and greater than or equal to 5 mm in length were the best cutoff values for the prediction of post-PCI thrombolysis in myocardial infarction (TIMI) flow grade less than 3.[9] The use of distal embolic protection should be considered for such high-risk lesions to decrease the incidence of no-reflow phenomenon and subsequent adverse cardiac events after PCI.[10]

Present IVUS measurements can also help operators identify optimal stent diameter and length.[11,12] Several potential approaches have been proposed for proper selection of stent diameter, including stent sizing based on the average lumen diameter of proximal and distal references, the smaller reference lumen diameter (usually the distal reference), and external elastic membrane (EEM) diameters at the lesion site. Midwall approach using the middle point between the lumen and EEM at the site of the minimal lumen diameter is another option for systematic stent sizing. Stent lengths are typically determined based on proximal and distal plaque burden. In general, angiographically normal reference site for PCI has plaque burden of 30% to 50% when assessed by IVUS.[13] Optimal landing zones are the segments with the least amount of plaque burden. If no segment has ideal plaque burden for the stent landing zone (<50% to 55%[14]), the site with the least available amount of plaque burden should be selected by IVUS.

Post-Stent Implantation

Following DES implantation, IVUS can visualize important findings related to stent failure.

Table 1 Intravascular ultrasonography checkpoints for stent optimization and stent failure		
Pre-PCI	**Post-PCI**	**Follow-up**
Stent sizing	Stent expansion	Neointimal hyperplasia
Stent length	Incomplete stent apposition	Tissue coverage
Prediction of stent underexpansion	Stent edge dissection	Stent fracture
Prediction of distal embolization	Tissue protrusion	Incomplete stent apposition
Need for plaque modification	Plaque burden at reference segments	Neoatherosclerosis

Abbreviation: PCI, percutaneous coronary intervention.

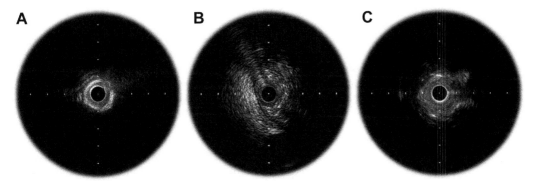

Fig. 1. Differential diagnosis of plaques with ultrasound signal dropout. (*A*) Calcified plaque with acoustic shadow: difficult to expand. (*B*) Attenuated plaque (eccentric, 0 to 4 o'clock): distal embolization (slow/no flow). (*C*) Attenuated plaque (all): distal embolization (slow/no flow).

Specifically, stent underexpansion, significant incomplete strut apposition (or malapposition) with impaired flow, residual plaque and/or dissection at stent edge, and extensive in-stent tissue protrusion have been considered as risk factors of stent failure. Among many IVUS criteria suggested for stent optimization, the first major IVUS-guided stent optimization strategy was the MUSIC (Multicenter Ultrasound Stenting in Coronaries Study) criteria proposed in the bare-metal stent era.[15] In the DES era, the AVIO (Angiography vs IVUS Optimization) study determined adjunctive balloon size by averaging the "media-to-media" diameters of distal and proximal stent segment, as well as at the site of narrowing within the stent.[16] Because stent underexpansion remains the main cause of DES failure, at least a minimal stent area (MSA) less than 5.0 mm^2 should be avoided in non–left main lesions.[17] Considering that the strict and universal criteria were infrequently achieved in the past clinical trials, a reasonable approach adoptable in daily clinical practice is to adjust the criteria for lesion types or to use relative cutoff values (Table 2).[18–20] In left main disease, for instance, the MSA cutoff value to predict subsequent stent failure was reported as 5.0 mm^2 for the ostial left circumflex, 6.0 mm^2 for the ostial left anterior descending, 7.0 mm^2 for the polygon of confluence, and 8.0 mm^2 for the left main artery.[21] In non–left main lesions treated with long stents, MSA greater than the distal reference lumen area was associated with a very low adverse clinical event rate (1.5% within 1 year).[19] With respect to the relative criteria, the optimal cutoff value of stent expansion to predict fractional flow reserve greater than 0.90 was reported as ~80%.[22]

Large stent edge dissection detected by IVUS has been reported to be associated with early stent thrombosis. In addition to its detection and association with residual plaque at the stent edge, IVUS can directly evaluate the depth and extension of the dissection, and major dissections (disrupting media or adventitia, or extensive lateral [>60°] and longitudinal extension [>2 mm]) should not be left untreated.[23] Recent development of high-resolution IVUS further improved the assessment of the dissections.[24,25]

Stent malapposition is defined as the lack of stent-vessel wall contact in at least 1 stent strut, not associated with a side-branch orifice. In a recent clinical study, acute stent malapposition was seen in 19% by post-PCI IVUS observation (14% major: 5% minor).[26] Although malapposition can resolve in time, it may also develop at follow-up at the segment where stent struts were initially in contact with the vessel wall at post-PCI, possibly as a result of underlying vascular inflammation and positive remodeling, predominantly seen in DES, or mural thrombus resolution after primary PCI with stenting in ACS lesions. Extensive acute stent malapposition should be avoided and corrected with postdilatation.

Table 2 Cutoff values of drug-eluting stent expansion	
	Minimal Stent Area
Recent generation drug-eluting stent (<28 mm)	≥5.0–5.5 mm^2
Long stent (≥28 mm)	≥5.0 mm^2 or ≥ distal reference lumen area
Left main coronary artery	≥8.0 mm^2
Relative cutoff values	≥90% of distal reference lumen area ≥80% of average reference lumen area

Tissue protrusion through stent struts is seen in 15% to 30% in chronic coronary syndrome and 50% to 70% in ACS.[27,28] Extensive tissue protrusion resulting in a small effective lumen area may cause early stent thrombosis in patients with ACS. Therefore, additional prolonged dilation with a postdilatation balloon can be used to crimp the protruded tissue to the wall, but it is important to keep the balloon size modest because of the risk of distal embolization.

POSSIBLE INTRAVASCULAR ULTRASOUND COMPLICATIONS AND TROUBLESHOOTING

The important complications associated with the use of IVUS are (1) transient ischemia, (2) coronary spasm, (3) air embolization, and (4) dissection of the coronary artery ostium. When IVUS is inserted into a tight stenosis and the observation time is prolonged, chest pain and ST-segment elevation on electrocardiography may occur.[29,30] For pre-PCI imaging, fast automated pullback may help minimize the ischemia caused by the imaging catheter insertion. If IVUS is difficult to pass through the lesion, predilation with a small-diameter balloon is recommended. To avoid coronary spasm, intracoronary nitrate should be administered before IVUS catheter insertion. If the air around the transducer is not fully removed when preparing, optimal IVUS images cannot be obtained. If flushes to clear the images are inadvertently performed within the coronary artery, air emboli can occur, causing transient slow flow and prolonged chest pain. Therefore, it is important to remove air bubbles while rotating the IVUS imaging core outside the body before IVUS insertion. When using a monorail-type IVUS catheter in chronic total occlusion (CTO) lesions, one should be aware that if the IVUS tip is trapped in a bending or calcified lesion during the catheter manipulation, the guiding catheter may be pulled into the coronary artery, potentially resulting in dissection of the coronary artery ostium.

Especially in lesions with strong bends, such as left circumflex and right coronary arteries, there is a possibility of entwining of the IVUS catheter and guidewire, or IVUS getting stuck in the distal portion of the stent. It is important to always return the imaging core to the tip after observation, keep rotating the transducer, and slowly retrieve the IVUS catheter while checking with fluoroscopy. In case of any resistance, the IVUS catheter should never be forcefully withdrawn further and bailout retrieval methods of the entrapped imaging catheter should be attempted.[31]

APPLICATIONS FOR SPECIFIC SITUATIONS
Left Main Lesions

It has been reported that the Medina classification on CAG does not correspond to the actual distribution of plaques on IVUS observation. In approximately 90% of cases, plaque is observed continuously from the left main coronary artery to the left anterior descending artery,[32] whereas plaque is infrequently observed on the flow divider. The advantages of IVUS guidance in PCI of bifurcation lesions include precise assessment of plaque distribution, prediction of side-branch occlusion, selection of appropriate stent type and size, prevention of inadequate stent expansion, malapposition, and stent deformation, and if indicated, assistance with plaque modification using atherectomy devices, all of which are critically important when treating the left main lesions.

As of today, the mainstream of bifurcation PCI with modern DES is the 1-stent strategy. In left main lesions, IVUS observation should be first performed to investigate lesion characteristics and plaque distribution. **Fig. 2** illustrates typical plaque distribution from the left main to the bifurcation. In the left main artery, plaque is often located in the contralateral portion of the carina (see **Fig. 2**A). If plaque is present in the direction of the side branch and extends to its entrance (see **Fig. 2**B) or if there is severe stenosis at the ostium of the side branch (see **Fig. 2**B, C), the risk of side-branch occlusion after stent placement is predicted to be high.[33] In this context, IVUS observation of the side branches plays a unique role because plaque may be present on IVUS even when there is no stenosis at the side-branch ostium on CAG. IVUS assessment of vessel and lumen diameters of the side branch also leads to precise selection of the optimal balloon size for side-branch dilation to prevent unfavorable side-branch dissection. When recrossing a guidewire into a jailed side branch after crossover stenting, the guidewire should be inserted through the most distal cell in the side-branch orifice possible. It is important to interpret the branch morphology in a three-dimensional manner and to ensure that as few struts as possible remain at the entrance of the side branch.[34]

Chronic Total Occlusions: Intravascular Ultrasound-Guided Wiring

Most CTOs are accompanied by side branches. In abrupt-type CTOs, IVUS is placed on the side branches to guide a high-penetration-force wire safely and securely into the plaque. In general, there are 2 typical PCI methods for CTO: the antegrade approach and the

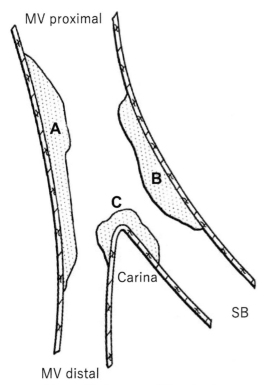

MV proximal

A

B

C

Carina

SB

MV distal

Fig. 2. Plaque distribution at bifurcation based on IVUS. (*A*) Plaque is present in the contralateral portion of the carina (MB). (*B*) Plaque is present in the direction of SB and extends to the entrance of SB. (*C*) Plaque is present on the carina side of SB. MB, main branch; SB, side branch.

retrograde approach. In the antegrade approach, the IVUS-guided CTO wiring is similar to the parallel wire technique. The direction in which the guidewire should be advanced can be determined based on the positional relationship between the IVUS catheter and the CTO wire. If the guidewire straying into the subintima is observed by IVUS, the guidewire is pulled out to the intimal area and then is advanced in a controlled direction toward the true lumen. At this procedure, the 3-dimensional wiring technique with angiography or IVUS guidance is useful. In the retrograde approach, the utility of IVUS is to identify the intravascular location of the retrograde guidewire as it passes through the CTO. IVUS inserted in an antegrade manner can resolve proximal cap ambiguity by CAG. In this application, a type of IVUS with a short distance from the tip to the transducer should be selected. IVUS can then provide useful information in sizing the balloon for reverse controlled antegrade retrograde tracking (CART), precisely adjusting the balloon placement, and confirming dissection formation.[35,36]

Calcified Lesions

In calcified lesions, pre-PCI imaging is important in determining the treatment strategy. In case of difficulty in advancing an IVUS catheter along the guidewire through the calcified lesion, a guide extension catheter may be useful.

Deep calcification often permits effective balloon dilation, whereas superficial calcification greater than a half circumference is expected to be difficult to dilate. If superficial calcifications are detected on IVUS but not recognized on CAG, the calcifications themselves are relatively thin and longitudinally confined, likely allowing sufficient dilatation.[37] In such lesions, use of a cutting/scoring balloon may facilitate creating a crack in the calcification. In circumferential napkin-ring-like calcified lesions, plaque modification with rotational atherectomy may be considered. Eccentric plaques with superficial calcification of greater than 180° but with the relatively normal contralateral wall are at high risk for coronary perforation (Fig. 3), and thus, modest balloon/stent sizing is recommended.

Although the efficacy of rotational atherectomy for severely calcified lesions is well established, it is important to predict complications specific to this procedure, such as coronary perforation and no-flow events. IVUS before the atherectomy is useful in understanding the position of the guidewire in relation to the vessel wall (guidewire bias), enabling operators to predict the exact location of calcium ablation. After rotational atherectomy, the location of the calcium ablation can be confirmed by a unique multiple reverberation appearance on postatherectomy IVUS.[38] One recent retrospective clinical study reported that the number of reverberations was also independently associated with the occurrence of slow flow phenomenon following rotational atherectomy, possibly reflecting the severity of calcifications such as the thickness and components.[39]

Diffuse Long Lesions

In diffuse long lesions, proper device sizing is particularly important for successful PCI. Pre-PCI IVUS can help evaluate the reference vessel diameter as well as the plaque characteristics and distribution to determine the optimal stent size and length.[40] Although full lesion coverage with DES is generally recommended, potential issues in this approach in diffuse long lesions, such as the increased risk of major side-branch encroachment or distal embolization due to the displacement of large amount of ASP, must be considered as well. If IVUS is used in manual mode, the projected stent landing sites should be coregistered with angiography by marking

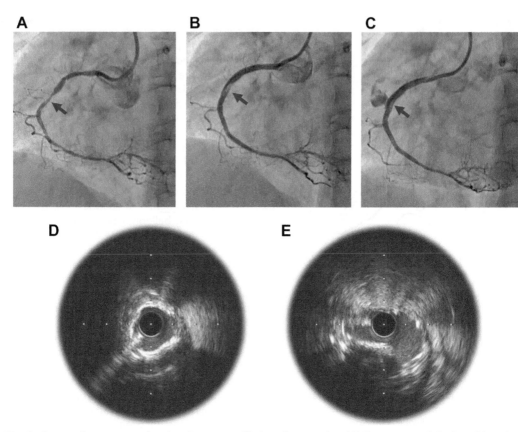

Fig. 3. A case of coronary perforation due to postdilation after stenting. (*A*) Severe stenosis in the midportion of the right coronary artery (RCA). (*B*) A 3.25 × 38-mm drug-eluting stent was implanted after predilatation. Angiographic haziness was observed in the lesion after the stenting. (*C*) Coronary perforation after postdilation with a 3.5 × 15 mm-noncompliant balloon. (*D*) IVUS image of the stenosis site showed 270° of severe calcification. (*E*) IVUS showed stent underexpansion (dot-to-dot indicates 1 mm). The red arrows in *A*, *B*, and *C* indicate the perforation site.

the IVUS transducer on the angiographic images (so-called marking technique) and the lesion length to be treated should be measured using the IVUS digital measure. The length of stent to be used is then determined according to this measured lesion length. In this context, it is essential to track precisely where the IVUS transducer is located in the target vessel.

In-Stent Restenosis

Despite robust use of IVUS to improve PCI outcomes, ISR remains even in the contemporary DES era. Other than the stent underexpansion and residual plaque at stent edge as the most commonly seen risk factors as described earlier, neoatherosclerosis may also be involved in the mechanism of ISR, and the timing and frequency of its occurrence have been reported to vary depending on the type of stents.[41] Other possible mechanisms include stent fracture,

polymer damage, and allergic reactions to polymers. Lesion-specific treatment strategy for ISR, such as plain balloon dilatation, drug-coated balloons, and additional stent, can be determined based on the exact mechanism revealed by intracoronary imaging findings.

Minimum-Contrast Percutaneous Coronary Intervention

Minimum-contrast PCI with IVUS is a technique to avert contrast nephropathy related to PCI procedure. In simple-lesion PCI, contrast volume can be adequately controlled when IVUS is fully used (ie, use IVUS to evaluate the lesion without contrast angiography, and stent the target lesion guided by IVUS transducer markings on fluorography).[42–44] Although it is often difficult to sufficiently control the amount of contrast media in complex-lesion PCI, information obtained with IVUS can help determine how to simplify

Table 3 Practical applications of intravascular ultrasonography	
Diagnostic use	1. Angiographically ambiguous lesions
	2. Left main coronary artery stenosis
	3. Complex bifurcation lesions
	4. Culprit lesions of acute coronary syndrome
PCI guidance and optimization	1. Long lesions
	2. Chronic total occlusions
	3. Acute coronary syndrome
	4. Left main lesions
	5. Complex bifurcation/ calcified lesions
	6. Renal dysfunction (reduce contrast media volume)

Abbreviation: PCI, percutaneous coronary intervention.

the PCI procedure. In practice, it is important to determine the safety limit for contrast usage. The target ratio of contrast volume to estimated glomerular filtration rate should be set to 1.0, and in case this is not feasible, a PCI strategy should be carefully planned so that the final ratio would not exceed 2.0.

SUMMARY

The clinical utility of IVUS for PCI guidance is now widely accepted, but the practical barriers to IVUS-guided PCI include extra cost, additional time for the imaging procedure, and training required for correct interpretation.[3,45] It is desirable to eliminate restrictions on the use of IVUS, but at least the most beneficial practical application would be for patients at greater risks of complications and restenosis (Table 3).[46] Although IVUS-derived complications, such as air bubble embolization and device entrapment, are rare, operators should be familiar with their causes and troubleshooting. Technical enhancements, such as lower profile catheter for better manipulation, faster pullback speed, higher resolution, IVUS-CAG coregistration, multimodality imaging catheters, and image interpretation/treatment planning assisted with artificial intelligence and machine learning, are evolving continuously, which may facilitate the clinical IVUS use by overcoming the current practical limitations in the near future.

CLINICS CARE POINTS

- The key question is how to use IVUS.
- To predict and prevent various complications, IVUS images should be thoroughly checked before and after stenting.
- Improving IVUS skills will further improve PCI outcomes.

CONFLICT OF INTEREST

The authors declare that they have no conflict of interest.

REFERENCES

1. Koskinas KC, Ughi GJ, Windecker S, et al. Intracoronary imaging of coronary atherosclerosis: validation for diagnosis, prognosis and treatment. Eur Heart J 2016;37:524–535a-c.
2. Mintz GS, Guagliumi G. Intravascular imaging in coronary artery disease. Lancet 2017;390:793–809.
3. Saito Y, Kobayashi Y, Fujii K, et al. Clinical expert consensus document on intravascular ultrasound from the Japanese Association of Cardiovascular Intervention and Therapeutics (2021). Cardiovasc Interv Ther 2022;37:40–51.
4. Mintz GS. Intravascular imaging of coronary calcification and its clinical implications. JACC Cardiovasc Imaging 2015;8:461–71.
5. Hoffmann R, Mintz GS, Popma JJ, et al. Treatment of calcified coronary lesions with Palmaz-Schatz stents. An intravascular ultrasound study. Eur Heart J 1998;19:1224–31.
6. Patel VG, Brayton KM, Mintz GS, et al. Intracoronary and noninvasive imaging for prediction of distal embolization and periprocedural myocardial infarction during native coronary artery percutaneous intervention. Circ Cardiovasc Imaging 2013;6:1102–14.
7. Pu J, Mintz GS, Biro S, et al. Insights into echo-attenuated plaques, echolucent plaques, and plaques with spotty calcification: novel findings from comparisons among intravascular ultrasound, near-infrared spectroscopy, and pathological histology in 2,294 human coronary artery segments. J Am Coll Cardiol 2014;63:2220–33.
8. Kimura S, Kakuta T, Yonetsu T, et al. Clinical significance of echo signal attenuation on intravascular ultrasound in patients with coronary artery disease. Circ Cardiovasc Interv 2009;2:444–54.
9. Endo M, Hibi K, Shimizu T, et al. Impact of ultrasound attenuation and plaque rupture as detected by intravascular ultrasound on the incidence of no-

reflow phenomenon after percutaneous coronary intervention in ST-segment elevation myocardial infarction. JACC Cardiovasc Interv 2010;3:540–9.

10. Hibi K, Kozuma K, Sonoda S, et al. A randomized study of distal filter protection versus conventional treatment during percutaneous coronary intervention in patients with attenuated plaque identified by intravascular ultrasound. JACC Cardiovasc Interv 2018;11:1545–55.

11. de Ribamar Costa J Jr, Mintz GS, Carlier SG, et al. Intravascular ultrasound assessment of drug-eluting stent expansion. Am Heart J 2007;153:297–303.

12. Cook S, Wenaweser P, Togni M, et al. Incomplete stent apposition and very late stent thrombosis after drug-eluting stent implantation. Circulation 2007;115:2426–34.

13. Mintz GS, Painter JA, Pichard AD, et al. Atherosclerosis in angiographically "normal" coronary artery reference segments: an intravascular ultrasound study with clinical correlations. J Am Coll Cardiol 1995;25:1479–85.

14. Sakurai R, Ako J, Morino Y, et al. Predictors of edge stenosis following sirolimus-eluting stent deployment (a quantitative intravascular ultrasound analysis from the SIRIUS trial). Am J Cardiol 2005;96: 1251–3.

15. de Jaegere P, Mudra H, Figulla H, et al. Intravascular ultrasound-guided optimized stent deployment. Immediate and 6 months clinical and angiographic results from the Multicenter Ultrasound Stenting in Coronaries Study (MUSIC Study). Eur Heart J 1998;19:1214–23.

16. Chieffo A, Latib A, Caussin C, et al. A prospective, randomized trial of intravascular-ultrasound guided compared to angiography guided stent implantation in complex coronary lesions: the AVIO trial. Am Heart J 2013;165:65–72.

17. Sonoda S, Morino Y, Ako J, et al. Impact of final stent dimensions on long-term results following sirolimus-eluting stent implantation: serial intravascular ultrasound analysis from the sirius trial. J Am Coll Cardiol 2004;43:1959–63.

18. Song HG, Kang SJ, Ahn JM, et al. Intravascular ultrasound assessment of optimal stent area to prevent in-stent restenosis after zotarolimus-, everolimus-, and sirolimus-eluting stent implantation. Catheter Cardiovasc Interv 2014;83:873–8.

19. Hong SJ, Kim BK, Shin DH, et al. Effect of intravascular ultrasound-guided vs angiography-guided everolimus-eluting stent implantation: the IVUS-XPL randomized clinical trial. JAMA 2015;314: 2155–63.

20. Lee SY, Shin DH, Kim JS, et al. Intravascular ultrasound predictors of major adverse cardiovascular events after implantation of everolimus-eluting stents for long coronary lesions. Rev Esp Cardiol (Engl Ed) 2017;70:88–95.

21. Kang SJ, Ahn JM, Song H, et al. Comprehensive intravascular ultrasound assessment of stent area and its impact on restenosis and adverse cardiac events in 403 patients with unprotected left main disease. Circ Cardiovasc Interv 2011;4:562–9.

22. Meneveau N, Souteyrand G, Motreff P, et al. Optical coherence tomography to optimize results of percutaneous coronary intervention in patients with non-ST-elevation acute coronary syndrome: results of the multicenter, randomized DOCTORS study (does optical coherence tomography optimize results of stenting). Circulation 2016;134:906–17.

23. Raber L, Mintz GS, Koskinas KC, et al. Clinical use of intracoronary imaging. Part 1: guidance and optimization of coronary interventions. An expert consensus document of the European Association of Percutaneous Cardiovascular Interventions. Eur Heart J 2018;39:3281–300.

24. Leesar MA, Saif I, Hagood KL, et al. A new method to optimize stent deployment by high-definition intravascular ultrasound. J Invasive Cardiol 2021; 33:E532–9.

25. Ando H, Nakano Y, Sawada H, et al. Diagnostic performance of high-resolution intravascular ultrasound for abnormal post-stent findings after stent implantation- a comparison study between high-resolution intravascular ultrasound and optical coherence tomography. Circ J 2021;85:883–90.

26. Ali ZA, Maehara A, Genereux P, et al. Optical coherence tomography compared with intravascular ultrasound and with angiography to guide coronary stent implantation (ILUMIEN III: OPTIMIZE PCI): a randomised controlled trial. Lancet 2016; 388:2618–28.

27. Qiu F, Mintz GS, Witzenbichler B, et al. Prevalence and clinical impact of tissue protrusion after stent implantation: an ADAPT-DES intravascular ultrasound substudy. JACC Cardiovasc Interv 2016;9: 1499–507.

28. Choi SY, Witzenbichler B, Maehara A, et al. Intravascular ultrasound findings of early stent thrombosis after primary percutaneous intervention in acute myocardial infarction: a Harmonizing Outcomes with Revascularization and Stents in Acute Myocardial Infarction (HORIZONS-AMI) substudy. Circ Cardiovasc Interv 2011;4:239–47.

29. Hausmann D, Erbel R, Alibelli-Chemarin MJ, et al. The safety of intracoronary ultrasound. A multicenter survey of 2207 examinations. Circulation 1995;91:623–30.

30. Batkoff BW, Linker DT. Safety of intracoronary ultrasound: data from a Multicenter European Registry. Cathet Cardiovasc Diagn 1996;38:238–41.

31. Hiraya D, Sato A, Hoshi T, et al. Incidence, retrieval methods, and outcomes of intravascular ultrasound catheter stuck within an implanted stent: systematic literature review. J Cardiol 2020;75:164–70.

32. Oviedo C, Maehara A, Mintz GS, et al. Intravascular ultrasound classification of plaque distribution in left main coronary artery bifurcations: where is the plaque really located? Circ Cardiovasc Interv 2010;3:105–12.

33. Furukawa E, Hibi K, Kosuge M, et al. Intravascular ultrasound predictors of side branch occlusion in bifurcation lesions after percutaneous coronary intervention. Circ J 2005;69:325–30.

34. de la Torre Hernandez JM, Baz Alonso JA, Gomez Hospital JA, et al. Clinical impact of intravascular ultrasound guidance in drug-eluting stent implantation for unprotected left main coronary disease: pooled analysis at the patient-level of 4 registries. JACC Cardiovasc Interv 2014;7:244–54.

35. Habara M, Tsuchikane E, Muramatsu T, et al. Comparison of percutaneous coronary intervention for chronic total occlusion outcome according to operator experience from the Japanese retrograde summit registry. Catheter Cardiovasc Interv 2016; 87:1027–35.

36. Sumitsuji S, Inoue K, Ochiai M, et al. Fundamental wire technique and current standard strategy of percutaneous intervention for chronic total occlusion with histopathological insights. JACC Cardiovasc Interv 2011;4:941–51.

37. Wang X, Matsumura M, Mintz GS, et al. In Vivo calcium detection by comparing optical coherence tomography, intravascular ultrasound, and angiography. JACC Cardiovasc Imaging 2017;10: 869–79.

38. Sakakura K, Yamamoto K, Taniguchi Y, et al. Intravascular ultrasound enhances the safety of rotational atherectomy. Cardiovasc Revasc Med 2018; 19:286–91.

39. Jinnouchi H, Sakakura K, Taniguchi Y, et al. Intravascular ultrasound-factors associated with slow flow following rotational atherectomy in heavily calcified coronary artery. Sci Rep 2022;12:5674.

40. Morino Y, Tamiya S, Masuda N, et al. Intravascular ultrasound criteria for determination of optimal longitudinal positioning of sirolimus-eluting stents. Circ J 2010;74:1609–16.

41. Nakazawa G, Otsuka F, Nakano M, et al. The pathology of neoatherosclerosis in human coronary implants bare-metal and drug-eluting stents. J Am Coll Cardiol 2011;57:1314–22.

42. Mariani J Jr, Guedes C, Soares P, et al. Intravascular ultrasound guidance to minimize the use of iodine contrast in percutaneous coronary intervention: the MOZART (Minimizing cOntrast utiliZation With IVUS Guidance in coRonary angioplasTy) randomized controlled trial. JACC Cardiovasc Interv 2014; 7:1287–93.

43. Ogata N, Ikari Y, Nanasato M, et al. Safety margin of minimized contrast volume during percutaneous coronary intervention in patients with chronic kidney disease. Cardiovasc Interv Ther 2014;29:209–15.

44. Ali ZA, Karimi Galougahi K, Nazif T, et al. Imaging- and physiology-guided percutaneous coronary intervention without contrast administration in advanced renal failure: a feasibility, safety, and outcome study. Eur Heart J 2016;37:3090–5.

45. Koskinas KC, Nakamura M, Raber L, et al. Current use of intracoronary imaging in interventional practice - Results of a European Association of Percutaneous Cardiovascular Interventions (EAPCI) and Japanese Association of Cardiovascular Interventions and Therapeutics (CVIT) Clinical Practice Survey. EuroIntervention 2018;14:e475–84.

46. Sonoda S, Hibi K, Okura H, et al. Current clinical use of intravascular ultrasound imaging to guide percutaneous coronary interventions. Cardiovasc Interv Ther 2020;35:30–6.

Intravascular Ultrasound-Guided Percutaneous Coronary Intervention: Evidence and Clinical Trials

Yong-Joon Lee, MD, Myeong-Ki Hong, MD*

KEYWORDS

• Percutaneous coronary intervention • Drug-eluting stent • Intravascular ultrasound

KEY POINTS

- Intravascular ultrasound (IVUS)-guided percutaneous coronary intervention (PCI) has shown benefits not only in patient with complex lesions but also in all-comers.
- The benefits of IVUS-guided PCI regarding clinical outcomes were maintained during the long-term follow-up.
- Further prospective confirmations especially regarding how to perform IVUS-guided PCI more efficiently are required to expand the use of IVUS during PCI in the real-world clinical practice.

INTRODUCTION

In the era of current interventional cardiology, percutaneous coronary intervention (PCI) with drug-eluting stent (DES) is widely performed in patients with even more complex coronary lesions than previously.[1–6] Intravascular imaging such as intravascular ultrasound (IVUS) provides detailed anatomic information during the PCI procedure.[3,4,7] During pre-intervention, detailed inspection for lesion characteristics such as lesion diameter, length, and plaque morphology is possible by using IVUS.[3,4,6,7] Based on this IVUS-based pre-intervention information, appropriate decision for stent size, length, and landing zone is possible.[3,4,6,7] Finally, during post-intervention, not only stent optimization with adequate stent expansion and full apposition of stent struts but also detection of procedural complications are possible with the help of IVUS which leads to improved post-procedural outcomes.[3,4,6,7] Along with the favorable procedural results by the use of IVUS, improved clinical outcomes after IVUS-guided PCI were shown in previous studies with long-term follow-up.[1,2,8,9] However, the use of IVUS during PCI remains low, therefore requires more efforts in order to strengthen the recommendations and consequently expand the use of IVUS in the real-world clinical practice.[3–6,10,11] The aim of this review is to discuss the previous evidences and clinical trials regarding IVUS-guided PCI and to discover the necessity for future studies to broaden its usage.

LESSONS FROM CLINICAL TRIALS

Benefit of Intravascular Ultrasound-Guided Percutaneous Coronary Intervention in Complex Lesions

Owing to the high cost and prolongation of the diagnostic procedure or intervention, IVUS was preferred in selective patients, especially in those with complex lesions.[10,11] The Angiography versus IVUS Optimization (AVIO) prospective, randomized, multicenter trial first evaluated the benefit of IVUS-guided PCI in DES era among patients with complex lesions (bifurcation, chronic total occlusion, long lesion, or small

Severance Hospital, Yonsei University College of Medicine, Seoul, South Korea
* Corresponding author. Division of Cardiology, Severance Hospital, Yonsei University College of Medicine, 50-1 Yonsei-ro, Seodaemun-gu, Seoul 03722, South Korea
E-mail address: mkhong61@yuhs.ac

Intervent Cardiol Clin 12 (2023) 177–185
https://doi.org/10.1016/j.iccl.2022.10.004
2211-7458/23/© 2022 Elsevier Inc. All rights reserved.

vessel).[12] Among 284 patients included in the trial, the post-intervention minimum lumen diameter was significantly larger in the IVUS-guided PCI compared with angiography-guided PCI (2.7 ± 0.5 mm vs 2.5 ± 0.5 mm, $P < .001$).[12] However, this trial was not powered enough to show significant difference in the rate of major adverse cardiac events (composite of cardiac death, myocardial infarction, or target-vessel revascularization) at 24 months, probably due to the limited number of study population.[12] The IVUS-XPL (Impact of Intravascular Ultrasound Guidance on Outcomes of Xience Prime Stents in Long Lesions) prospective, randomized, multicenter trial first demonstrated the benefit of IVUS-guided PCI regarding clinical outcomes among patients requiring DES implantation for long coronary lesion, compared with angiography-guidance.[1] Long coronary lesion was defined as implanted stent ≥28 mm in length and 1400 patients were enrolled.[1] During the 12-month follow-up, the rate of composite of major adverse cardiac events (composite of cardiac death, target-lesion-related myocardial infarction, or ischemia-driven target-lesion revascularization) was significantly lower in the IVUS-guided PCI, compared with angiography-guided PCI (2.9% vs 5.8%; hazard ratio [HR]: 0.48; 95% confidence interval [CI]: 0.28–0.83; $P = .007$).[1] The benefit of IVUS-guided PCI was mainly driven by a lower risk of target-lesion revascularization (2.5% vs 5.0% HR: 0.51, 95% CI: 0.28–0.91, $P = .02$).[1] The CTO-IVUS (Chronic Total Occlusion Intervention with Drug-eluting stents guided by IVUS) prospective, randomized, multicenter trial first presented the benefit of using IVUS in chronic total occlusion intervention.[13] Among 402 patients enrolled in the trial, IVUS-guided PCI significantly improved the rate of major adverse cardiac events rate (composite of cardiac death, myocardial infarction, or target-vessel revascularization) at 12 months, as compared with angiography-guidance (2.6% vs 7.1%, HR: 0.35, 95% CI: 0.13–0.97, $P = .035$).[13] The benefit of using IVUS in left main disease intervention was demonstrated by de la Torre Hernandez and colleagues in their patient-level pooled data of four registries regarding left main disease treated with DES with 505 matched pairs of IVUS-or angiography-guided PCI.[14] During the 36-month follow-up, the rate of major adverse events (composite of cardiac death, myocardial infarction, or target-lesion revascularization) was significantly lower in the IVUS-guided PCI, as compared with angiography-guided PCI (11.7% vs 16.0%, $P = .04$).[14] Consistent results were found in a meta-analysis based

on three randomized trial including 2345 patients treated with DES for complex lesions.[15] The rate of major adverse cardiac events (composite of cardiac death, myocardial infarction, or stent thrombosis) at 12 months was significantly lower in the IVUS-guided PCI compared with angiography-guided PCI (0.4% vs 1.2%; HR: 0.36; 95% CI: 0.13–0.99; $P = .040$).[15] Similarly, based on their institutional registry, Choi and colleagues demonstrated the advantage of IVUS-guided PCI in large number of patients with various complex lesions including bifurcation, chronic total occlusion, left main, long lesion, multivessel PCI, multiple stent implantation, in-stent restenosis, or heavily calcified lesions.[16] Among 6005 patients undergoing PCI for complex lesions, IVUS was used in 1674 patients (27.9%).[16] During the median follow-up of 64 months, IVUS-guided PCI was associated with lower rate of major adverse cardiac events (composite of cardiac death, myocardial infarction, ischemia-driven target-lesion revascularization, or stent thrombosis) compared with angiography-guidance (18.5% vs 28.1%, HR: 0.63, 95% CI: 0.53–0.73, $P < .001$). Based on these studies, IVUS has been recommended in patients with necessity, especially in those with complex lesions.[3–5]

Benefit of Intravascular Ultrasound-Guided Percutaneous Coronary Intervention in All-Comers

Although the benefits of IVUS-guided PCI in patients with complex lesions were shown with evidences, the potential benefit of IVUS-guidance in all-comer patients including not only with complex lesions but also with simple lesions was unclear.[1,13–16] The Assessment of Dual Antiplatelet Therapy with Drug-Eluting Stents (ADAPT-DES) study was a prospective, nonrandomized, multicenter study of 8583 all-comer patients and among the study population, 3349 patients (39%) underwent DES implantation with IVUS-guidance.[17] IVUS-guided PCI was associated with lower rate of composite of major adverse cardiac events (composite of cardiac death, myocardial infarction, or stent thrombosis) at 12 months, compared with angiography-guidance (3.1% vs 4.7%; adjusted HR: 0.70; 95%; CI: 0.55–0.88; $P = .002$).[17] The ULTIMATE (Intravascular Ultrasound Guided Drug Eluting Stents Implantation in All-Comers Coronary Lesions) trial was the first prospective, randomized, multicenter trial which demonstrated the benefit of IVUS-guided PCI in all-comers undergoing DES implantation.[2] The only lesion characteristics to be excluded in the trial were chronic total occlusion or severely calcified lesion requiring rotational atherectomy.[2] During the 12-month follow-up, the rate of target-vessel failure (composite of cardiac death, target-vessel myocardial infarction, or clinically driven target-vessel revascularization) was significantly lower in the IVUS-guided PCI compared with angiography-guidance (2.9% vs 5.4%; HR: 0.53; 95% CI: 0.31–0.90; $P = .019$).[2] The benefit of IVUS-guided PCI was mainly driven by a lower risk of target-vessel revascularization (1.5% vs 2.9% HR: 0.51, 95% CI: 0.25–1.07, $P = .07$).[2] It is notable that the results of the ULTIMATE trial were similar to those of IVUS-XPL, which specifically focused on the patients requiring DES implantation for long lesions.[1,2] Consistent results were found in a meta-analysis based on 31 studies including 17,882 patients.[18] The risks of all-cause death (odds ratio [OR]: 0.74%; 95% credible interval [CrI]: 0.58–0.98), myocardial infarction (OR: 0.72%; 95% CrI: 0.52–0.93), target-lesion revascularization (OR: 0.74%, 95% CrI: 0.58–0.90), and stent thrombosis (OR: 0.42%; 95% CrI: 0.20–0.72) were significantly lower in the IVUS-guided PCI compared with angiography guidance.[18] The trend and benefit of using IVUS in all-comers was demonstrated by Mentias and colleagues, based on the US Medicare cohort of 1,877,177 patients including 105,787 patients (5.6%) who underwent IVUS-guided PCI.[11] The use of IVUS during PCI increased from 3.0% in 2009 to 6.9% in 2017 (P for trend <0.01).[11] Compared with angiography-guidance, IVUS-guided PCI was associated with lower rate of 12-month mortality (12.3% vs 11.5%, $P < .001$), myocardial infarction (5.2% vs 4.9%, $P < .001$), and repeat revascularization (6.7% vs 6.1%, $P < .001$).[11] The results were consistent not only in long-term follow-up which will be discussed in detail in the following issue but also in all subgroups of stent type (bare metal stent or DES), clinical presentation (stable coronary artery disease or acute coronary syndrome), procedural complexity (complex PCI or noncomplex PCI), and facility of IVUS utilization (moderate [1%–5%], frequent [5%–10%], or very frequent use of IVUS [>10%]).[11] Although the use of IVUS is limited by expenses, procedural time, and varied across hospitals, it has shown benefits in various patients and lesions, therefore, more efforts to encourage the use of IVUS are required to improve the clinical outcomes after PCI.[1,2,10,11,13–18] A summary of the prospective studies regarding IVUS-guided PCI versus angiography-guidance is presented in Table 1.

Long-Term Follow-Up After Intravascular Ultrasound-Guided Percutaneous Coronary Intervention

Whether the beneficial effect of IVUS-guided PCI versus angiography-guidance is sustained beyond 1 year has been reported, most noticeably from IVUS-XPL and ULTIMATE trials.[8,9] In IVUS-XPL trial which focused on the patients requiring DES implantation for long lesions, 1183 patients (85%) completed 5-year follow-up, and the rate of composite of major adverse cardiac events at 5 years was significantly lower in the IVUS-guided PCI compared with angiography-guidance (5.6% vs 10.7%; HR: 0.50; 95% CI: 0.34–0.75; $P = .001$).[1,8] The difference was mainly driven by lower risk of target-lesion revascularization, and the sustained clinical benefits were from not only within first 1 year but also from 1 to 5 year after PCI. Similarly, in ULTIMATE trial which included all-comer patients requiring DES implantation, 1423 patients (98.3%) completed 3-year follow-up, and the rate of target-vessel failure at 3 years was significantly lower in the IVUS-guided PCI compared with angiography-guidance (6.6% vs 10.7%; HR: 0.60; 95% CI: 0.42–0.87; $P = .01$), mainly driven by lower risk of target-vessel revascularization.[2,9]

Although the benefit of IVUS-guided PCI during long-term follow-up was reported in IVUS-XPL and ULTIMATE trials, these two trials included repeat revascularization in the primary outcomes and the benefits of using IVUS with regard to primary outcomes were principally driven by a reduction in the need for repeat revascularization rather than a reduction in mortality.[1,2,8,9] Furthermore, no difference was observed in each trial regarding the occurrence of hard clinical outcomes such as composite of cardiac death, myocardial infarction, or stent thrombosis. Recently, from the patient-level pooled data of these two trials, Hong and colleagues reported the long-term benefit of IVUS-guided PCI regarding hard clinical outcomes in 2577 patients with long lesions treated with DES (implanted stent length ≥ 28 mm).[19] During the 3-year follow-up, the rate of cardiac death was significantly lower in the IVUS-guided PCI compared with angiography-guidance (1.0% vs 2.2%; HR: 0.43; 95% CI: 0.22–0.84; $P = .011$).[19] Furthermore, the rate of composite of cardiac death, myocardial infarction, or stent thrombosis was significantly lower in the IVUS-guided PCI (1.3% vs 2.9%; HR: 0.44; 95% CI: 0.25–0.80; $P = .005$).[19] The long-term benefit of IVUS-guided PCI regarding

Table 1
Representative prospective studies regarding intravascular ultrasound-guided percutaneous coronary intervention versus angiography-guidance

Study (Year of Publication)	Randomized	Number of Patients IVUS-Guidance	Angiography-Guidance	Study Population	Follow-up (Months)	Primary Outcome	Results
AVIO (2013)	Randomized	142	142	Patients with complex lesions (bifurcation, long lesion, chronic total occlusion, or small vessel)	24	Post-intervention minimum lumen diameter	Superior in IVUS-guided PCI (2.7 ± 0.5 mm vs 2.5 ± 0.5 mm, $P < .001$), however failed to show superiority in 24-mo clinical outcomes
ADAPT-DES (2014)	Nonrandomized	3349	5234	All-comers	12	Definite/probable stent thrombosis	Superior in IVUS-guided PCI (3.1% vs 4.7%, $P < .002$)
CTO-IVUS (2015)	Randomized	201	201	Patients with chronic total occlusion	12	Cardiac death	Failed to show superiority in IVUS-guided PCI (0% vs 1.0%, $P = .16$), however superiority was shown regarding composite of cardiac death, myocardial infarction, or target-vessel revascularization
IVUS-XPL (2015)	Randomized	700	700	Patients with long lesion (implanted stent length ≥28 mm)	12	Major adverse cardiac events (composite of cardiac death, myocardial infarction, or target-lesion revascularization)	Superior in IVUS-guided PCI (2.9%. vs 5.8%, $P = .007$)
ULTIAMTE (2018)	Randomized	724	724	All-comers	12	Target-vessel failure (composite of cardiac death, myocardial infarction, or target-vessel revascularization)	Superior in IVUS-guided PCI (2.9% vs 5.4%, $P = .019$)

Abbreviations: ADAPT-DES, assessment of dual antiplatelet therapy with drug-eluting stents; AVIO, angiography versus IVUS optimization; CTO-IVUS, chronic total occlusion intervention with drug-eluting stents guided by IVUS; IVUS, intravascular ultrasound; IVUS-XPL, impact of intravascular ultrasound guidance on outcomes of Xience Prime Stents in long lesions; PCI, percutaneous coronary intervention; ULTIMATE, intravascular ultrasound guided drug eluting stents implantation in all-comers coronary lesions.

hard clinical outcomes was also noted in the US Medicare cohort-based study.[11] During the median follow-up of 3.7 years, IVUS-guided PCI was associated with lower rate of all-cause death (82.8 vs 88.7 event per 1000 person-years; adjusted HR: 0.92; 95% CI: 0.91–0.94; $P < .001$) and myocardial infarction (33.5 vs 35.8 events per 1000 person-years; adjusted HR: 0.93; 95% CI: 0.90–0.95; $P < .001$) compared with angiography-guidance.[11] The longer follow-up results were demonstrated by Choi and colleagues in patients who underwent PCI for various complex lesions based on their institutional registry.[16] During the median follow-up of 5.3 years, IVUS-guided PCI was associated with lower rate of all-cause death (10.2% vs 16.9%; HR: 0.57; 95% CI: 0.46–0.71; $P < .001$), myocardial infarction (4.8% vs 7.3%; HR: 0.64; 95% CI: 0.48–0.86; $P = .003$), and stent thrombosis (3.1% vs 4.4%; HR: 0.60; 95% CI: 0.41–0.86; $P = .006$) compared with angiography-guidance.[16] The 10-year follow-up results from the IVUS-XPL and ULTIMATE trials are greatly expected.

Intravascular Ultrasound-Defined Stent Optimization Criteria

After stent deployment, IVUS can detect abnormalities such as stent under-expansion, malapposition, and edge dissection which may hinder achieving optimal results after PCI.[3,4,6] In IVUS-XPL trial, stent optimization was defined as minimum stent area (MSA) greater than the distal reference lumen area on IVUS, and meeting IVUS-defined stent optimization was associated with lower rate of composite of major adverse cardiac events at 12 months compared with not meeting optimization (1.5% vs 4.6%; HR: 0.31: 95% CI: 0.11–0.86; $P = .02$).[1] In ULTIMATE trial, more strict criteria for stent optimization were adopted which required that all three of following criteria be met: (1) MSA greater than 5.0 mm^2 or 90% of the distal reference lumen area; (2) plaque burden 5 mm proximal or distal to the stent edge less than 50%; and (3) no edge dissection involving the media with length more than 3 mm on IVUS.[2] Meeting IVUS-defined stent optimization was associated with a lower rate of the target-vessel failure at 12 months compared with not meeting optimization (1.6% vs 4.4%; HR: 0.35: 95% CI: 0.14–0.90; $P = .029$), and the results were consistent during 3-year follow-up (4.2% vs 9.2%; HR: 0.44: 95% CI: 0.24–0.81; $P = .01$).[2,9] Therefore, efforts are required to improve the correctable abnormalities noted on IVUS to achieve optimal results after stent implantation.[3,4,6]

Adequate stent expansion has been considered as most consistent parameter to predict adverse clinical outcomes after DES implantation, which expansion criteria to adopt in clinical practice still a highly controversial topic.[3,4] Although previous IVUS studies have been showing that an MSA of 5.5 mm^2 best discriminated subsequent adverse events, these studies have primarily focused on angiographic restenosis or repeat revascularization with short-term follow-up.[3,4,20,21] On the other hand, in the subanalysis of ADAPT-DES study, 10 different stent expansion criteria were evaluated for predicting composite of definite stent thrombosis or clinically driven target-lesion revascularization at 2 years (Table 2).[22] Among the 10 stent expansion criteria, only MSA/vessel area at MSA site was independently associated with composite of definite stent thrombosis or target-lesion revascularization (adjusted HR: 0.77; 95% CI: 0.59–0.99; $P = .04$).[22] Recently, the long-term effect of seven different absolute or relative expansion criteria for IVUS-defined optimal stent expansion regarding hard clinical outcome (composite of cardiac death, target-lesion related myocardial infarction, or stent thrombosis) was evaluated in 1254 patients who underwent IVUS-guided DES implantation to treat a long lesion (implanted stent length ≥28 mm) from the pooled data of IVUS-XPL and ULTIMATE trials (see Table 2).[23] The rate of 3-year hard clinical outcome was lower in patients with optimal stent expansion compared with those without optimal stent expansion according to only three criteria: MSA greater than 5.5 mm^2 (0.5% vs 2.2%; HR: 0.21; 95% CI: 0.06–0.75; $P = .008$), MSA greater than 5.0 mm^2 (0.6% vs 2.6%; HR: 0.24; 95% CI: 0.09–0.68; $P = .003$), and MSA/distal reference lumen area greater than 90% (0.5% vs 2.4%; HR: 0.32; 95% CI: 0.12–0.88; $P = .019$).[23] Achieving other relative expansion criteria was not associated with a reduction in hard clinical outcome.[23] Furthermore, the notable finding was that even with the use of IVUS, achieving optimal stent expansion of MSA greater than 5.5 mm^2, greater than 5.0 mm^2, or MSA/distal reference lumen area greater than 90% was possible only in 51.4%, 65.6%, and 65.2% of procedures, which raises the issue of more effective way of using IVUS and more devotional effort to achieve optimal expansion.[23] The reason for different findings found in the subanalysis of ADAPT-DES study and pooled analysis of IVUS-XPL and ULTIMATE trials may be due to different criteria applied and different study population; therefore, further prospective

Table 2
Summary of studies regarding intravascular ultrasound-defined optimal stent expansion

	Subanalysis of ADAPT DES	Pooled Analysis of IVUS-XPL and ULTIMATE
Number of patients	1831	1254
Study population	All-comers	Patients with long lesion (implanted stent length ≥28 mm)
Expansion criteria	1) MSA 2) MSA/vessel area at MSA site 3) MSA/average reference lumen area 4) Minimum stent expansion using Huo-Kassab model 5) Minimum stent expansion by linear model accounting for vessel tapering 6) Stent asymmetry (minimum/maximum stent diameter within the entire stent) 7) Stent eccentricity (smallest minimum/maximum stent diameter at a single slice within the stent) 8) IVUS-XPL criteria[a] 9) ULTIMATE criteria[b] 10) ILUMIEN IV criteria[c]	Absolute optimal expansion criteria 1. MSA > 5.5 mm^2 2. MSA > 5.0 mm^2 Relative optimal expansion criteria 1. MSA/distal reference lumen area >100% 2. MSA/distal reference lumen area >90% 3. MSA/distal reference lumen area >80% 4. MSA/average reference lumen area >90% 5. MSA/average reference lumen area >80%.
Follow-up (months)	24	36
Primary outcome	Composite of definite stent thrombosis or clinically driven target-lesion revascularization	Composite of cardiac death, target-lesion-related myocardial infarction, or stent thrombosis
Results	Among the 10 stent expansion criteria, only MSA/vessel area at MSA site was independently associated with lower rate of primary outcome.	Among the 7 stent expansion criteria, only MSA >5.5 mm^2, MSA >5.0 mm^2, and MSA/distal reference lumen area >90% were associated with significantly lower rate of primary outcome.

Abbreviations: ADAPT-DES, assessment of dual antiplatelet therapy with drug-eluting stents; IVUS, intravascular ultrasound; IVUS-XPL, impact of intravascular ultrasound guidance on outcomes of Xience Prime Stents in long lesions; MSA, minimum stent area; ULTIMATE, intravascular ultrasound guided drug eluting stents implantation in all-comers coronary lesions.
[a] Defined as MSA greater than the distal reference lumen area.
[b] Defined as MSA greater than 5.0 mm^2 or greater than 90% of distal reference lumen area.
[c] Defined as MSA of the proximal segment ≥90% of proximal reference lumen area and MSA of the distal segment ≥90% of distal lumen reference area.

confirmation is warranted to confirm which optimal stent expansion criteria to adopt in clinical practice.

Stent Optimization Using Intravascular Ultrasound

Although post-dilation after DES implantation is frequently performed to achieve optimal stent expansion and full apposition of stent struts, the specifics while performing post-dilation such as final balloon size and inflation pressure are highly dependent on the operator; therefore, the effect of post-dilation on clinical outcomes is conflicting.[7,24] On the other hand, IVUS can detect stent under-expansion that cannot be easily identified by angiography and consequently motivate more effective post-dilation with the appropriate size and inflation pressure of the balloons.[7,22] In ADAPT-DES study, when IVUS was used during PCI, the

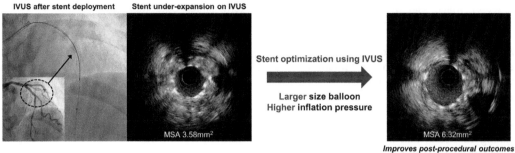

IVUS after stent deployment   Stent under-expansion on IVUS

Stent optimization using IVUS

Larger size balloon
Higher inflation pressure

MSA 3.58mm²

MSA 6.32mm²

*Improves post-procedural outcomes
and long-term clinical outcomes*

Fig. 1. Effective post-dilation using IVUS after stent deployment. After stent deployment, IVUS can detect stent under-expansion which cannot be easily identified by angiography, therefore more effective post-dilation can be performed using larger size balloon with higher inflation pressure. In this representative case, MSA was successfully increased from 3.58 to 6.32 mm² after IVUS-guided post-dilation. IVUS, intravascular ultrasound; MSA, minimum stent area.

operator changed the PCI strategy in 74% of the patients to choose a larger devices (38%), higher inflation pressure (23%), and additional post-dilation (13%).[17] Similarly, among patients who underwent DES implantation for complex lesions, IVUS-guided PCI was associated with a more frequent use of post-dilation compared with angiography-guidance (49.0% vs 17.9%; $P < .001$).[16] Recently, the effect of IVUS-guided post-dilation and angiography-guided post-dilation was evaluated compared with angiography-guided DES implantation without post-dilation as a reference, among the patients who underwent IVUS-guided DES implantation to treat a long lesion (implanted stent length $\geq$28 mm) from the pooled data of IVUS-XPL and ULTIMATE trials.[25] More effective post-dilation was performed in IVUS-guided post-dilation group using a larger size balloon (3.6 ± 0.7 mm vs 3.5 ± 0.6 mm; $P < .001$) and higher maximum inflation pressure (18.7 ± 4.1 atm vs 18.2 ± 4.1 atm; $P = .005$) compared with angiography-guided post-dilation.[25] Consequently, although post-intervention minimum lumen diameter was significantly larger in the IVUS-guidance with post-dilation group versus the angiography-guidance without post-dilation (2.6 ± 0.5 mm vs 2.5 ± 0.4 mm; $P = .046$), it was not different between the angiography-guidance with post-dilation group versus the angiography-guidance without post-dilation (2.5 ± 0.4 mm vs 2.5 ± 0.4 mm; $P = .367$).[25] This may indicate that the use of IVUS should be encouraged throughout the procedure not only during pre-intervention and stent selection but also after stent deployment to obtain optimal results after DES implantation. Park and colleagues proposed the concept of intracoronary imaging-

guided pre-dilation, stent sizing, and post-dilation (iPSP) strategy to improve clinical outcomes in patients with complex lesions.[7] From the Interventional Cardiology Research In-cooperation Society Drug-Eluting Stents registry, among 9525 patients undergoing DES implantation to treat complex lesion (left main, bifurcation, long, or severely calcified lesion), 3374 patients (35.4%) underwent DES implantation applying all 3 components of the iPSP strategy.[7] Using iPSP strategy was associated with significantly lower rate of primary outcome (composite of cardiac death, target-vessel myocardial infarction, or target-vessel revascularization) at 3 years compared with not using the strategy (5.6% vs 7.9%; adjusted HR: 0.71; 95% CI 0.63–0.81; $P < .001$).[7] However, among the three components of iPSP strategy, post-dilation was only independently associated with lower risk of primary outcome which may be due to effective post-dilation using larger final balloon size.[7] Representative example of effective post-dilation using IVUS after stent deployment is presented in Fig. 1. Beyond merely using IVUS during PCI, more effective way of using it is necessary, and therefore requires further prospective confirmation regarding iPSP strategy and each component of the strategy.

FURTHER STUDIES EXPECTED

Recently, the deep-learning approach has been widely applied in medical imaging which can develop predictive model with excellence performance. Min and colleagues reported a deep-learning algorithm based on pre-intervention IVUS images and clinical information (stent diameter, length, and inflation pressure; balloon diameter; and maximal balloon pressure) which can accurately predict stent under-expansion (accuracy 94% and area under the curve 0.94).[26] Further studies regarding the IVUS image-based data-driven approach may assist physicians in making treatment decision to achieve optimal results after DES implantation.

Despite limited with high expenses, longer procedural time, and requirement for proper training to obtain and interpret images, IVUS-guided PCI has shown benefit in patients with complex lesions as well as simple lesions.[1–4,10,13–15,18] Furthermore, the benefit was sustained during the long-term follow-up.[8,9,11,16] The on-going DKCRUSH VIII (IVUS-guided DK Crush Stenting Technique for Patients With Complex Bifurcation Lesions) trial (NCT03770650) comparing IVUS-guided PCI versus angiography-guidance in systemic two-stent strategy for treating complex bifurcation lesion and IMPROVE (IMPact on Revascularization Outcomes of IVUS Guided Treatment of Complex Lesions and Economic Impact) trial (NCT04221815) comparing IVUS-guided PCI versus angiography-guidance in various complex lesions are expected to expand the use of IVUS in the era of DES. Furthermore, the details regarding IVUS-guided PCI such as IVUS-defined stent optimization criteria, iPSP strategy, and post-dilation using IVUS that was associated with improved clinical outcomes in previous studies should be further evaluated through prospective, randomized, controlled trials.

CLINICS CARE POINTS

- Intravascular ultrasound (IVUS)-guided percutaneous coronary intervention (PCI) has shown benefits in patient with complex lesions.

- The benefits of IVUS-guided PCI were also present in all-comer patients.

- The benefits of IVUS-guided PCI were maintained during the long-term follow-up.

- The details regarding IVUS-defined stent optimization require further prospective confirmations.

SUMMARY

The IVUS-guided PCI that was associated with improved post-procedural outcomes and long-

term clinical outcomes has shown benefits in patients with complex lesions as well as simplex lesions. However, the use of IVUS during PCI remains low; therefore, further prospective, randomized, controlled trials especially regarding how to perform IVUS-guided PCI more efficiently are required to strengthen the recommendations and consequently broaden its use in the real-world clinical practice.

DISCLOSURE

None.

CONFLICT OF INTEREST

None.

REFERENCES

1. Hong SJ, Kim BK, Shin DH, et al. Effect of Intravascular Ultrasound-Guided vs Angiography-Guided Everolimus-Eluting Stent Implantation: The IVUS-XPL Randomized Clinical Trial. JAMA 2015; 314(20):2155–63.

2. Zhang J, Gao X, Kan J, et al. Intravascular Ultrasound Versus Angiography-Guided Drug-Eluting Stent Implantation: The ULTIMATE Trial. J Am Coll Cardiol 2018;72(24):3126–37.

3. Räber L, Mintz GS, Koskinas KC, et al. Clinical use of intracoronary imaging. Part 1: guidance and optimization of coronary interventions. An expert consensus document of the European Association of Percutaneous Cardiovascular Interventions. Eur Heart J 2018;39(35):3281–300.

4. Maehara A, Matsumura M, Ali ZA, et al. IVUS-Guided Versus OCT-Guided Coronary Stent Implantation: A Critical Appraisal. J Am Coll Cardiol Img 2017;10(12):1487–503.

5. Neumann FJ, Sousa-Uva M, Ahlsson A, et al. 2018 ESC/EACTS Guidelines on myocardial revascularization. Eur Heart J 2019;40(2):87–165.

6. Mintz GS, Guagliumi G. Intravascular imaging in coronary artery disease. Lancet 2017;390(10096): 793–809.

7. Park H, Ahn JM, Kang DY, et al. Optimal Stenting Technique for Complex Coronary Lesions: Intracoronary Imaging-Guided Pre-Dilation, Stent Sizing, and Post-Dilation. J Am Coll Cardiol Intv 2020;13(12):1403–13.

8. Hong SJ, Mintz GS, Ahn CM, et al. Effect of Intravascular Ultrasound-Guided Drug-Eluting Stent Implantation: 5-Year Follow-Up of the IVUS-XPL Randomized Trial. J Am Coll Cardiol Intv 2020; 13(1):62–71.

9. Gao XF, Ge Z, Kong XQ, et al. 3-Year Outcomes of the ULTIMATE Trial Comparing Intravascular Ultrasound Versus Angiography-Guided Drug-Eluting

Stent Implantation. J Am Coll Cardiol Intv 2021; 14(3):247–57.

10. Koskinas KC, Nakamura M, Räber L, et al. Current use of intracoronary imaging in interventional practice - Results of a European Association of Percutaneous Cardiovascular Interventions (EAPCI) and Japanese Association of Cardiovascular Interventions and Therapeutics (CVIT) Clinical Practice Survey. EuroIntervention 2018;14(4):e475–84.

11. Mentias A, Sarrazin MV, Saad M, et al. Long-Term Outcomes of Coronary Stenting With and Without Use of Intravascular Ultrasound. J Am Coll Cardiol Intv 2020;13(16):1880–90.

12. Chieffo A, Latib A, Caussin C, et al. A prospective, randomized trial of intravascular-ultrasound guided compared to angiography guided stent implantation in complex coronary lesions: the AVIO trial. Am Heart J 2013;165(1):65–72.

13. Kim BK, Shin DH, Hong MK, et al. Clinical Impact of Intravascular Ultrasound-Guided Chronic Total Occlusion Intervention With Zotarolimus-Eluting Versus Biolimus-Eluting Stent Implantation: Randomized Study. Circ Cardiovasc Interv 2015;8(7): e002592.

14. de la Torre Hernandez JM, Baz Alonso JA, Gómez Hospital JA, et al. Clinical impact of intravascular ultrasound guidance in drug-eluting stent implantation for unprotected left main coronary disease: pooled analysis at the patient-level of 4 registries. J Am Coll Cardiol Intv 2014;7(3):244–54.

15. Shin DH, Hong SJ, Mintz GS, et al. Effects of Intravascular Ultrasound-Guided Versus Angiography-Guided New-Generation Drug-Eluting Stent Implantation: Meta-Analysis With Individual Patient-Level Data From 2,345 Randomized Patients. J Am Coll Cardiol Intv 2016; 9(21):2232–9.

16. Choi KH, Song YB, Lee JM, et al. Impact of Intravascular Ultrasound-Guided Percutaneous Coronary Intervention on Long-Term Clinical Outcomes in Patients Undergoing Complex Procedures. J Am Coll Cardiol Intv 2019;12(7):607–20.

17. Witzenbichler B, Maehara A, Weisz G, et al. Relationship between intravascular ultrasound guidance and clinical outcomes after drug-eluting stents: the assessment of dual antiplatelet therapy with drug-eluting stents (ADAPT-DES) study. Circulation 2014;129(4):463–70.

18. Buccheri S, Franchina G, Romano S, et al. Clinical Outcomes Following Intravascular Imaging-Guided Versus Coronary Angiography-Guided Percutaneous Coronary Intervention With Stent Implantation: A Systematic Review and Bayesian Network Meta-Analysis of 31 Studies and 17,882 Patients. J Am Coll Cardiol Intv 2017;10(24):2488–98.

19. Hong SJ, Zhang JJ, Mintz GS, et al. Improved Three-Year Cardiac Survival After IVUS-guided Long DES Implantation: A Patient-Level Analysis from Two Randomized Trials. J Am Coll Cardiol Intv (in press).

20. Hong MK, Mintz GS, Lee CW, et al. Intravascular ultrasound predictors of angiographic restenosis after sirolimus-eluting stent implantation. Eur Heart J 2006;27(11):1305–10.

21. Doi H, Maehara A, Mintz GS, et al. Impact of post-intervention minimal stent area on 9-month follow-up patency of paclitaxel-eluting stents: an integrated intravascular ultrasound analysis from the TAXUS IV, V, and VI and TAXUS ATLAS Workhorse, Long Lesion, and Direct Stent Trials. J Am Coll Cardiol Intv 2009;2(12):1269–75.

22. Fujimura T, Matsumura M, Witzenbichler B, et al. Stent Expansion Indexes to Predict Clinical Outcomes: An IVUS Substudy From ADAPT-DES. J Am Coll Cardiol Intv 2021;14(15):1639–50.

23. Lee YJ, Zhang JJ, Mintz GS, et al. Impact of Intravascular Ultrasound-Guided Optimal Stent Expansion on 3-Year Hard Clinical Outcomes. Circ Cardiovasc Interv 2021;14(10):e011124.

24. Romagnoli E, Sangiorgi GM, Cosgrave J, et al. Drug-eluting stenting: the case for post-dilation. J Am Coll Cardiol Intv 2008;1(1):22–31.

25. Lee YJ, Zhang JJ, Mintz GS, et al. Is routine post-dilation during angiography-guided stent implantation as good as intravascular ultrasound-guidance? An analysis using data from IVUS-XPL and ULTIMATE. Circ Cardiovasc Interv (in press).

26. Min HS, Ryu D, Kang SJ, et al. Prediction of Coronary Stent Underexpansion by Pre-Procedural Intravascular Ultrasound-Based Deep Learning. J Am Coll Cardiol Intv 2021;14(9):1021–9.

Intravascular Ultrasound and Optical Coherent Tomography Combined Catheter

Shigetaka Kageyama, MD[a], Nozomi Kotoku, MD[a],
Kai Ninomiya, MD[a], Shinichiro Masuda, MD[a],
Jiayue Huang, MSc[a], Takayuki Okamura, MD, PhD[b],
Scot Garg, MD, PhD[c], Isao Mori, MS[d],
Brian Courtney, MD[e], Faisal Sharif, MD, PhD[a],
Christos V. Bourantas, MD, PhD[f,g],
Patrick W. Serruys, MD, PhD[a],
Yoshinobu Onuma, MD, PhD[a,*]

KEYWORDS

- Combined catheter • Intravascular ultrasound • Optical coherent tomography
- Percutaneous coronary intervention • Coronary artery disease

KEY POINTS

- Intravascular ultrasound (IVUS) has high tissue penetration for assessing the entire coronary arterial wall.
- Optical coherence tomography (OCT) has a higher resolution to assess endoluminal structures.
- Combined IVUS-OCT probes work in synergy.

▶ **Video content accompanies this article at** http://www.interventional.theclinics.com.

INTRODUCTION

History and Background

Intravascular imaging was first developed to differentiate between abnormal and normal coronary arteries in vitro and in vivo. The first device was intravascular ultrasound (IVUS), which was introduced by Yock and colleagues in the 1980s[1] with its initial application to examine "whether the vessel was healthy or not by checking that the 3 layers of the artery were visible." Optical coherence tomography (OCT) was introduced in the 1990s as a second type of intravascular imaging tool, which could "evaluate vascular tissues with higher resolution"[2,3] with the first-in-man OCT

study conducted in 2002.[4] The concept behind both devices is similar in terms of visualizing intra-coronary structures by reconstructing images from signal waves scattered by the vessel wall; however, disparities in signal utilization (ultrasound [frequency 20–60 MHz] in IVUS and low-coherence light [wavelength 1.3 μm] in OCT[5]) characterize the differences between the 2 technologies, especially in scan depth and resolution.

The resolution with OCT is higher than all other contemporary coronary imaging modalities (axial 10–20 μm and lateral 20–90 μm), and notably, it is approximately 10 times greater than that of IVUS (axial 100–150 μm and lateral

[a] Department of Cardiology, National University of Ireland, Galway (NUIG), University Road, Galway H91 TK33, Ireland; [b] Division of Cardiology, Department of Medicine and Clinical Science, Yamaguchi University Graduate School of Medicine, Yamaguchi, Japan; [c] Department of Cardiology, Royal Blackburn Hospital, Blackburn, UK; [d] Terumo Corporation, Tokyo, Japan; [e] Schulich Heart Program, Sunnybrook Research Institute, University of Toronto, Toronto, Ontario, Canada; [f] Department of Cardiology, Barts Heart Centre, Barts Health NHS Trust, London, UK; [g] Institute of Cardiovascular Sciences University College London, London, UK
* Corresponding author.
E-mail address: yoshinobu.onuma@nuigalway.ie

Intervent Cardiol Clin 12 (2023) 187–201
https://doi.org/10.1016/j.iccl.2022.12.002
2211-7458/23/© 2023 Elsevier Inc. All rights reserved.

150–300 μm).[6] Consequently, compared with IVUS, OCT can provide more detailed assessment of the lumen level and of superficial plaque (eg, in detecting plaque erosion, plaque rupture, and thin cap fibro atheroma [TCFA]) while also enabling clearer identification of suboptimal percutaneous coronary intervention (PCI) results such as coronary dissections, tissue protrusions, stent under expansion, and stent strut malapposition.[7] Long-term follow-up with OCT can evaluate the neointimal proliferation, neoatherosclerosis, uncovered struts, persistent/late-acquired stent malapposition, and/or coronary evagination, which could all be associated with adverse events.[8–10] Ultrasound is significantly influenced by the presence of calcium; calcified plaque reflects ultrasound signal, and therefore, the evaluation of plaque behind calcium is not feasible by IVUS.[11] However, with OCT, calcified plaques are recognized as low-intensity structures with clear demarcation of the calcific tissue borders.[12] However, OCT has a lower tissue penetration depth (1–2 mm) than IVUS (5–6 mm), which limits OCT imaging, particularly in the presence of highly attenuating structures such as red thrombus or lipid/necrotic core.[6] In this context, unlike OCT, IVUS enables assessment of the deeper layers of the vessel including the external elastic membrane.

The advantages and disadvantages of IVUS and OCT are listed in Table 1. Besides differences in penetration depth and resolution, there are also technical differences between the two. A priming-free catheter is available in optical frequency domain imaging (OFDI), which contributes to a shortened setup time; the pullback speed of OCT is more than twice that of IVUS; and OCT requires additional contrast injections to eliminate red blood cells.

Intravascular imaging is more suitable for assessing atherosclerosis in coronary arteries compared with luminography using angiography not only in terms of quantifying the severity of stenoses but also in terms of quantifying and characterizing plaque, especially when using IVUS. For example, we can evaluate stenosis, positive remodeling, and plaque characteristics at the same time. Foremost, the basic principle for assessing lesions using intravascular imaging is different to quantitative coronary angiography (QCA) (Fig. 1).[13] In QCA, percent diameter stenosis is calculated as (interpolated reference diameter [IRD] – minimal lumen diameter)/IRD, whereas the percent plaque area at the minimal lumen area (MLA) site obtained by intravascular imaging is calculated as (external elastic membrane area – lumen area)/external elastic membrane area.[14,15] Fig. 1 illustrates that the discrepancy in plaque size calculated from the IRD (dotted line) can occur either due to the incorrect assumption as to the start of the stenosis or due to outward expansion of plaque caused by focal compensatory enlargement.

The clinical applications of intravascular imaging have evolved during 35 years and now include (1) a research tool for investigating the progression and regression of coronary artery disease (CAD) with or without drug interventions, (2) qualitative and quantitative assessment of vulnerable plaque, and (3) guiding the indication for PCI and guiding the PCI procedure including sizing of devices, and optimization of the treated lesion.

Both intracoronary technologies have been validated against histology and are clinically relevant to prognosis as mentioned above.[16,17] The fundamental differences in imaging physics between IVUS and OCT result in different information being obtained, and thus a combination of these technologies potentially results in a synergistic improvement in the assessment of coronary atherosclerosis. Consequently, combined catheters have been developed that make the most of the advantages of each device and compensate for their deficiencies.

The Latest Recommendations in the Guidelines

In the latest European Society of Cardiology guidelines as well as the updated American College of Cardiology/American Heart Association guidelines, OCT use for stent optimization has a class IIa recommendation, which is on par with the recommendations for IVUS.[18,19] The guidelines were upgraded in 2021 to reflect several RCTs, observational studies and meta-analysis that have shown improved outcomes with intravascular imaging, such as reduced ischemic events. It should be acknowledged that the majority of the data in the literature still emanates from IVUS-related studies but the guidelines acknowledge that OCT can be used instead of IVUS in certain situations, such as non-ostial lesions and the absence of significant renal insufficiency. The Japanese Circulation Society guideline gives IVUS use a class I recommendation, especially for PCI of the left main stem and chronic total occlusions.[20]

COMBINED IMAGING TECHNOLOGY

The Rationale for Intravascular Ultrasound/Optical Coherence Tomography Combined Catheter

The accuracy of assessing tissue composition of atherosclerotic lesions varies between IVUS and

Table 1 Advantages and disadvantages of the intravascular ultrasound and optical coherent tomography		
	Advantage	**Disadvantage**
IVUS	• No contrast media needed • Aorto ostial evaluation is possible • Deep penetration depth	• Low pullback speed (1–9 mm/s) • Low resolution (not suitable for 3D reconstruction) • Acoustic shadow behind dense calcification
OCT	• High pullback speed (20 mm/s) • High resolution (suitable for 3D reconstruction and judging precise stent apposition) • Enable to measure the thickness of calcium	• Need to inject contrast media but can be replaced by low-molecular dextran • Not suitable for aorto ostial scan • Shallow depth of penetration • Attenuation behind red thrombus and lipid pool

Abbreviations: IVUS, intravascular ultrasound; OCT, optical coherent tomography.

OCT, and therefore, a combined approach is expected to further enhance diagnostic precision (agreement between OCT and histology κ = 0.67, IVUS and histology κ = 0.33).[21] Indeed, Li and colleagues[22] reported a high correlation between plaque circumference percent derived from the IVUS-OCT combined catheter compared with histology. In addition, perfect coregistration of IVUS and OCT images is a big advantage of the combined catheter. Räber and colleagues[23] first reported the offline fusion of IVUS and OCT images; however, the major limitation of their methodology was that the fusion was obtained from a sequential assessment using 2 separate probes, which is time-consuming, expensive, and theoretically less reproducible (Fig. 2).

Although the catheter profile is slightly larger than single image modalities, the feasibility of the combined catheter has already been proven in human coronary arteries.[24] A combined IVUS–OCT catheter system is warranted to enable accurate online coregistration and fusion of high-quality images obtained by the 2 imaging probes during a single pullback.

The Development of Combined Catheter and Its Advantages

IVUS and OCT have evolved in parallel during the last few years, and only recently have combined IVUS-OCT systems been developed to merge the advantages of both modalities into a single catheter.[25–27] The first combined IVUS–OCT catheter was designed by Li and colleagues[25] and Yin and colleagues[27] and was tested in a healthy rabbit aorta; however, the prototype had a 7.2Fr diameter, which made it unsuitable for clinical use. In 2011, Yin and colleagues reported a modified combined miniaturized OCT–IVUS probe,[28] which had an outer

diameter of 3.6Fr. achieved by arranging the position of the OCT and IVUS probe sequentially, followed in 2012 by the sequential probe system, which allowed more accurate coregistration,[29] and then in 2013 a back-to-back arrangement of the IVUS–OCT probe,[30] which had a higher frame rate of 20 fps compared with earlier models. In 2015, Li and colleagues[31] performed an ex vivo run of an advanced IVUS–OCT prototype (72fps) using postmortem human coronary arteries. In 2018, the first clinical use of the combined IVUS–OCT catheter was reported by Sheth and colleagues,[24] showing coregistered images with clinically acceptable specifications for size, speed, and resolution. Even though the catheter profile is slightly thicker than the latest single catheter, a combined catheter compensates for the disadvantages of a single modality in both de novo lesions and lesions after stent implantation (Figs. 3–5).[32,33]

Update of Currently Available Intravascular Ultrasound-Optical Coherence Tomography Combined Catheters

We report on the status of 2 IVUS-OCT combined catheter systems (CONAVI and TERUMO) together with showing some of their latest images.[33] In addition, a Chinese company, Panovision is preparing a first-in-man trial of a novel IVUS-OCT combined catheter; however, the details are unknown.[34]

CONAVI: the Novasight Hybrid System

The Novasight Hybrid System was developed by Conavi Medical Inc. (Toronto, Canada) and researchers at the University of Toronto.

The catheter is compatible with a 0.014-inch guidewire and has a 1.7 Fr. tip, a 2.8 Fr. distal imaging window, and a 3.3 Fr. catheter shaft. A colinear imaging design with overlapping

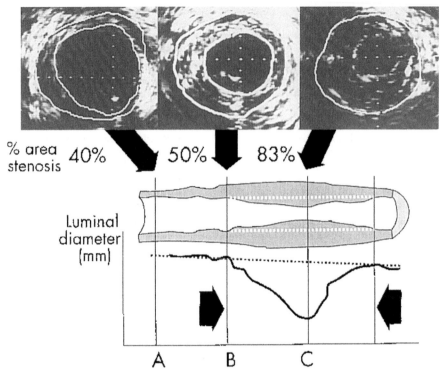

% area stenosis 40% 50% 83%

Luminal diameter (mm)

A   B   C

Fig. 1. Differences in the measurement of diameter stenosis in QCA and area stenosis in IVUS. IVUS, intravascular ultrasound; QCA, quantitative coronary angiography. (*Data from* Escaned et al. Significance of automated stenosis detection during quantitative angiography. Insights gained from intracoronary ultrasound imaging. Circulation. 1996;94(5):966-972.)

IVUS and OCT (Fig. 6) allows the user to visualize the vessel wall with both modalities simultaneously and inherently acquire accurate coregistered images. Lumen or vessel size can be measured using both IVUS and OCT cross-sectional images.

Pullback speeds between 0 and 25 mm/s can be selected with a maximum pullback length of 100 mm. In the case of standalone IVUS imaging, the frame rate is 30 or 100 fps. In the case of combined IVUS and OCT imaging, the pullback will be performed at 100 fps after blood clearance. The system does not allow the acquisition of only OCT. The maximum field of view radius is 6 mm derived from IVUS.

The first clinical use of Novasight was reported by Sheth and colleagues, in 2018,[35] wherein the system provided colocalized IVUS and OCT images of a nonculprit left anterior descending (LAD) artery in a patient with a recent ST-segment elevation MI. Lipid-rich plaques, bifurcations, and deeply embedded tissues were more clearly identified by IVUS images than OCT, whereas calcifications, stent struts, and fine dissections were more clearly identified by OCT imaging. The Novasight system is currently Food and Drug Administration (FDA) 510(k) cleared and has Health Canada approval. A prospective observational study using the catheter has been completed and demonstrated its feasibility and efficacy for diagnostic purposes, and for guiding PCI in 20 patients with chronic or acute coronary syndromes (ACS) (NCT03484975). The latest pullback images from the in vivo trial are available in Video 1.

TERUMO: the Dual Sensor

The Dual Sensor IVUS–OCT catheter system was developed by TERUMO (Tokyo, Japan) by merging IVUS and OFDI probes, which are already clinically available and incorporated in the AltaView (PMDA approval) and FastView (PMDA and CE mark approval), respectively.

Imaging is acquired with a sequential arrangement of an IVUS transducer and an optical lens (Fig. 7). The catheter is compatible with a 0.014-inch guidewire and has a diameter of 2.6 Fr. (3.0 Fr. catheter shaft).

The IVUS probe has an axial resolution of 120 µm, whereas the OCT has an axial resolution of 20 µm. The high frame rate (maximum 160 fps) permits a change in the pullback speed of up to 40 mm/s and a study length of up to

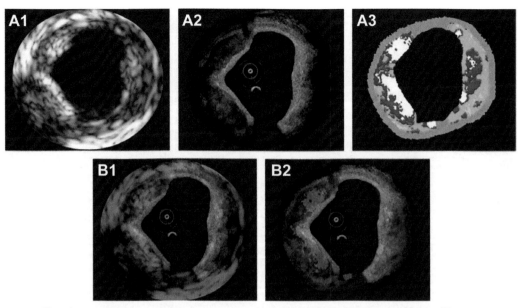

Fig. 2. Offline fusion of IVUS and OCT images. In panels, A$_{1-3}$ matched cross-sections obtained by IVUS-GS (A$_1$), OCT (A$_2$), and IVUS-VH (A$_3$) depict fibrocalcific plaque in the left half of the vessel, and a necrotic core/lipid pool at the opposite side of the calcification. Superimposing IVUS-GS on top of OCT and IVUS-VH on top of OCT is presented in panels B$_1$ and B$_2$, respectively. IVUS-GS, gray-scale intravascular ultrasound; IVUS-VH, virtual histology intravascular ultrasound. (*Data from* Räber et al. Offline fusion of co-registered intravascular ultrasound and frequency domain optical coherence tomography images for the analysis of human atherosclerotic plaques. EuroIntervention 2012;8:98-108.)

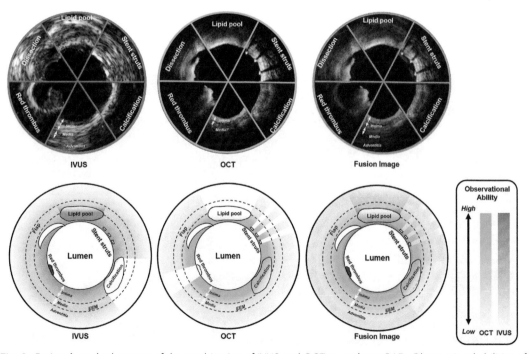

Fig. 3. Rationale and advantage of the combination of IVUS and OCT to evaluate CAD. Observational abilities of IVUS and OCT in the settings of several intracoronary structures. These colocalized images were obtained from the latest evaluation of the de novo coronary artery by Novasight Hybrid. IVUS, intravascular ultrasound; OCT, optical coherent tomography.

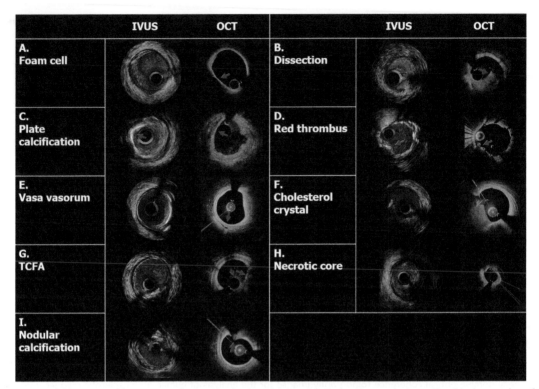

Fig. 4. Advantages and limitations of intravascular imaging modalities in de novo lesions. Graphical summary of the ability of IVUS of OCT and of the combined IVUS-OCT imaging in assessing de novo coronary artery characteristics and identifying features associated with future events. *Red arrows* indicate the points where each finding is located. IVUS, intravascular ultrasound; OCT, optical coherent tomography.

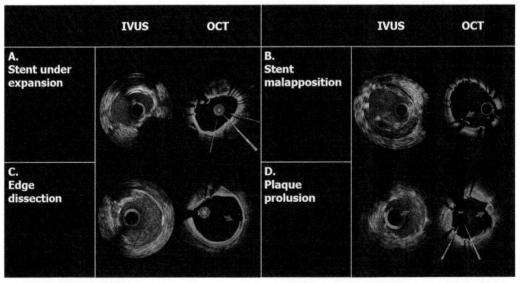

Fig. 5. Advantages and limitations of intravascular imaging modalities in stent implantation. Graphical summary of the ability of IVUS of OCT and of the combined IVUS-OCT imaging in assessing PCI results and identifying features associated with future events. *Red arrows* indicate the points where each finding is located. IVUS, intravascular ultrasound; OCT, optical coherent tomography.

150 mm. The acquired images can project side by side or as one fused image (see Fig. 9). Integrated-backscatter IVUS (IB-IVUS) analysis is also available, providing further information about tissue and plaque characteristics (Fig. 8).

Online OFDI 3D reconstruction facilitates a comprehensive evaluation of complex coronary artery structures. The device has been tested in postmortem coronary arteries, and its output was compared with the colocalized pathological specimens (Video 2). In this combined catheter, IVUS or OCT can be used together or separately. Operators can select an imaging modality according to procedural requirements. For instance, in the left main coronary artery (LMCA) disease, the operator can use this function to select IVUS to assess the severity and guide treatment strategy, with OCT used to assess the results of treatment including stent apposition and/or bifurcation optimization.

Potential Clinical Applications of a Combined Intravascular Ultrasound-Optical Coherence Tomography Catheter and Future Perspectives

Intravascular tool to evaluate regression or progression of the coronary plaque and vascular inflammation in natural history and pharmacotherapy

Intravascular imaging devices have been used to investigate the natural history of coronary plaque progression and the effect of lipid-lowering drugs on reducing plaque volume. Fig. 9 shows the correlation between achieved LDL-C levels and the median change in percent atheroma volume (PAV) and demonstrates the concordant and additive effects of high-intensity statins and PCSK-9 inhibitors on plaque regression.[36,37]

Using grayscale IVUS, the SATURN study showed that statin therapy is more effective in preventing plaque progression in high-risk patients with greater baseline coronary atheroma volume.[38] Kataoka and colleagues[39] reported that in patients with stable CAD and high-risk plaque, nonstatin use was associated with accelerated atheroma progression in nonculprit segments, whereas atheroma regression was observed with statins. In the GLAGOV trial, IVUS demonstrated a greater decrease in PAV in the group treated with evolocumab in addition to statins at 18-month follow-up.[40] In the ESCORT study, Akasaka and colleagues[41] used OCT to demonstrate that early statin therapy reduces TCFAs. In the PACMAN-AMI trial multimodality imaging was used to assess vulnerable plaque more accurately with 3

intravascular imaging modalities, including the near-infrared spectroscopy (NIRS)-IVUS combined catheter, used in every participant: PAV via IVUS, fibrous cap thickness via OCT, and lipid burden via NIRS.[42]

Atherosclerosis is a chronic inflammatory disease of the arterial wall and the effectiveness of statins, PCSK9 inhibitors, and other drugs targeting the immune system for treating atherosclerosis have been proven in several trials (eg, Canakinumab Anti-Inflammatory Thrombosis Outcome Study [CANTOS], COLchicine Cardiovascular Outcomes Trial [COLCOT], and Low-Dose Colchicine [LoDoCo] trial).[43–46] In addition, more and more trials are running to examine the impact of novel anti-inflammatory drugs.[43] In contemporary practice, most vascular inflammation is assessed using fluorodeoxyglucose PET-CT; however, the combined IVUS-OCT catheter could be an alternative if it could evaluate plaque volume and characterize plaque, together with assessing vascular inflammation at the same time. This would also be beneficial in terms of cost-effectiveness, especially for the secondary prevention population.

Intravascular tool for vulnerable plaque detection (demote)

The combined catheter is expected to compensate for the disadvantages and amplify the advantages of the single catheter and detect vulnerable plaque more accurately.

In 1989, James Muller first proposed the concept of vulnerable plaque,[47] and 18 years later, a consensus document of definitions, classifications, and clinical pathological evaluations was published.[48,49] Major criteria of vulnerable plaque are active inflammation, a thin cap with a large lipid core, endothelial denudation with superficial platelet aggregation, fissured/injured plaque, and severe stenosis.

It has been proved by various studies that intravascular imaging is useful to assess vulnerable plaque. The PROSPECT study demonstrated that a large plaque burden ($\geq$70%) and TCFA detected by IVUS-radiofrequency (RF) as well as a minimal lumen area less than 4.0 mm^2 were independent predictors of major adverse cardiac events (MACE) in nonculprit lesions of patients with ACS.[50] The Integrated Biomarkers and Imaging Study (IBIS) IV trial showed that high-intensity statin reduced RF-IVUS-defined atherosclerosis in noninfarct-related arteries among patients with myocardial infarction (MI).[51] The LRP study was the first prospective large-scale imaging study that examined the efficacy of NIRS-IVUS in detecting vulnerable

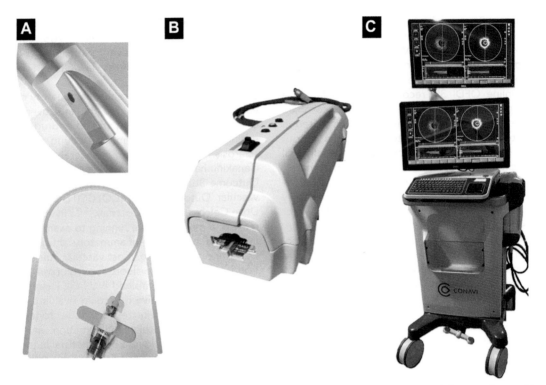

Fig. 6. CONAVI Novasight Hybrid imaging catheter; external appearances. (*A*) Catheter and the transducer with colinear arrangement. (*B*) Interface module. (*C*) A whole appearance of the system body. IVUS, intravascular ultrasound; OCT, optical coherence tomography.

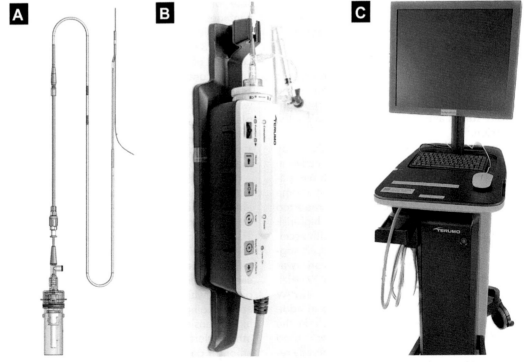

Fig. 7. TERUMO The Dual Sensor combined imaging catheter; external appearances. (*A*) Catheter technical specifications. (*B*) Interface module. (*C*) A whole appearance of the system body. IVUS, intravascular ultrasound; OCT, optical coherence tomography.

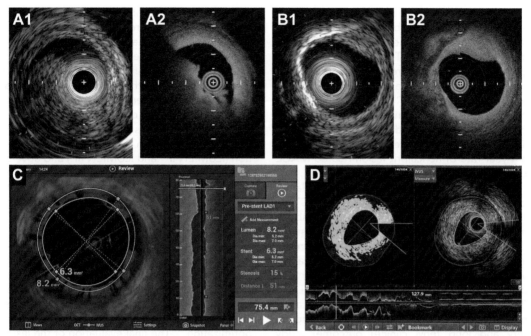

Fig. 8. IVUS, OCT, and fusion images obtained from TERUMO The Dual Sensor. TERUMO combined IVUS–OCT catheter system; sample images. (A) Coregistered intracoronary imaging of thrombus in IVUS (A₁) and OCT (A₂) in a cadaver coronary artery. (B) Coregistered intracoronary imaging of calcification in IVUS (B₁) and OCT (B₂) in a cadaver coronary artery. (C) Fusion image of IVUS and OCT. (D) IB-IVUS image with gray-scale IVUS. IB, integrated backscatter; IVUS, intravascular ultrasound; OCT, optical coherence tomography. (*Data from* Ono et al. Advances in IVUS/OCT and Future Clinical Perspective of Novel Hybrid Catheter System in Coronary Imaging. Front Cardiovasc Med. 2020;7:119.)

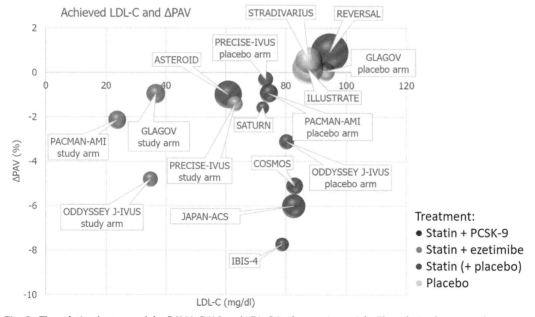

Fig. 9. The relation between delta PAV (ΔPAV) and LDL-C in the previous trials. The relation between plaque progression or regression (ΔPAV) and LDL-C values at the endpoint compared with the baseline. The mean value of ΔPAV and LDL-C was pointed in each treatment arm of the trials. ΔPAV, delta percent atheroma volume; LDL-C, low-density lipoprotein cholesterol.

plaques on a lesion level. The study enrolled 1241 patients with stable angina (46.3%) or ACS (53.7%) and assessed more than 5000 lesions with NIRS-IVUS.[52] The lesion-level analysis demonstrated that the presence of lipid-rich plaque (LCBI$_{4mm}$ > 400) was associated with a 4-fold higher event rate. PROSPECT II trial showed having one or more lesions with both a large plaque burden as detected by IVUS and a large lipid-rich core as detected by NIRS resulted in a 4-year rate of nonculprit lesion-related MACE of 13.2%.[53]

With the advantage of high resolution, plaque characterization is more detailed with OCT. In the recent COMBINE OCT-FFR study of diabetic patients with intermediate lesions, the presence of TCFA was associated with a 4.7-fold increase in the primary endpoint of cardiac death, target vessel MI, target lesion revascularization, or hospitalization for angina.[54] Recently, the CLIMA (Relationship between Coronary pLaque morphology of the left anterIor descending artery and long terM clinicAl outcome) study demonstrated that OCT-defined plaque vulnerability features (MLA <3.5 mm^2, TCFA, lipid arc circumferential extension >180, and macrophage findings) in the LAD were significantly associated with the increased risk of a composite of cardiac death and target-segment MI at 12 months among patients undergoing clinically indicated coronary angiography.[55]

The combined catheter enables the evaluation of the plaque burden assessed by IVUS and the vulnerability assessed by OCT such as TCFA, which may increase the precision of the prediction of future events.[5] In addition, the recent advance in the software enables the assessment of the OCT or IVUS-derived fractional flow reserve (FFR), which could be used as a surrogate for the wire-based FFR and potentially allow comprehensive assessment in plaque characteristics and ischemia in one pullback. It would remain as a question of whether the combined catheter could show incremental value to the currently available imaging modality, NIRS-IVUS.

Adjunctive imaging for procedure guidance

In current guidelines for revascularization, the use of IVUS or OCT to optimize stent implantation has a class IIa recommendation in select patients, especially in those with complex lesions.[18–20]

Various trials have shown the benefit of intravascular imaging in improving prognosis after PCI. IVUS-XPL trial,[56,57] the AVIO trial,[58] and the ULTIMATE[59,60] support the use of IVUS as a tool to guide PCI in contemporary practice. The treatment of bifurcation lesions is improved using intravascular imaging; the OPTIMUM trial showed online 3-dimension OFDI was superior to angiography-guidance only in terms of acute stent apposition at the bifurcation,[61] whereas the LEMON study demonstrated the feasibility of OCT-Guided PCI of the LMCA.[62] Head-to-head comparison trials of IVUS and OCT showed comparable results in terms of stent optimization (ILUMIEN II[63] and ILUMIEN III[7]) and adverse cardiac events (OPINION trial[64]).

Combined IVUS–OCT catheters have the potential to support procedures with high diagnostic efficacy derived from the combination of the 2 imaging modalities. For example, in the LMCA disease, which involves both aorto-ostial lesion and bifurcation lesion, the indication of PCI in the entire lesion can be assessed by IVUS. To facilitate the procedure, OCT will be used in each step of the intervention like recrossing the wire to the jailed side branch and stent optimization.[61] The final evaluation of the lesion is preferable to be done by OCT in terms of high resolution; however, IVUS alone could be relied on if there are concerns about renal function and total amount of contrast media. By using a combined catheter, we can use each modality or both modalities considering the situation of diagnosis and intervention as well as lesion location comprehensively.

Other Combined Catheters

Apart from the IVUS-OCT combined catheter, several other imaging modalities have been developed: NIRS-IVUS has already been mentioned while intravascular photoacoustic (IVPA) imaging, near-infrared fluorescence (NIRF) molecular imaging, time-resolved fluorescence spectroscopy (TRFS), and fluorescence lifetime imaging (FLIm) all provide additional information about plaque morphology and pathobiology.[65,66] Based on the same concept of developing the IVUS-OCT combined catheter, multimodalities were merged for their complementary strengths (Table 2).

So far, only the combined NIRS-IVUS catheter has been used clinically. In 2008, a single NIRS system was developed (LipiScan, Infraredx Inc., Bedford, MA, USA) and received FDA approval. Subsequently, a dual-modality system, which combined IVUS with NIRS, was developed (TVC Imaging System and Makoto Intravascular Imaging System, Infraredx Inc.) and received its CE mark in 2010. The device was used in the previously mentioned LRP, PROSPECT II, and PACMAN-AMI clinical trials.[67] A prototype

Table 2
Variations of combined catheters and their advantages

		OCT		IVUS	
	Axial Resolution	8 μm		20 μm	
OCT	8 μm	—		Detailed plaque characterization with vessel size (remodeling) assessment	
NIRS	NA	Differentiating deep tissue (ie, deeply embedded calcific tissue and lipid tissue)		Simultaneous assessment of lipid component and vessel structure (plaque burden, remodeling). Only combined catheter clinically applied	
NIRF	NA	Correlates inflammation and detailed morphological assessment		Simultaneous assessment of Inflammation and vessel structure	
IVPA	100 μm	—		Simultaneous assessment of chemical composition (ie, lipid, inflammation, stent) and structural information	
TRFS	160 μm	—		Simultaneous assessment of compositional characteristics (ie, lipid, collagen, elastin) of the superficial plaque and vessel structure	
FLIm	NA	Simultaneous assessment of compositional characteristics (ie, low-density lipoprotein, collagen, elastin) of the superficial plaque[a]		—	

Abbreviations: FLIm, fluorescence lifetime imaging; IVPA, intravascular photoacoustic imaging; IVUS, intravascular ultrasound; NIRF, near-infrared fluorescence; NIRS, near-infrared spectroscopy; OCT, optical coherent tomography; TRFS, time-resolved fluorescence spectroscopy.

[a] The image was cited from Kim S et al. Comprehensive Assessment of High-Risk Plaques by Dual-Modal Imaging Catheter in Coronary Artery. JACC Basic Transl Sci. 2021;6(12):948-960.

OCT-NIRS catheter has also been developed by the team at Massachusetts General Hospital and the first tests performed on autopsy specimens showed promising results. SpectraWAVE Inc. is preparing a commercial combination OCT-NIRS catheter, which was initially planned to be available for clinical use in 2021.[68]

LIMITATIONS

Despite the effort of industry and clinicians, the development of combined catheters has been slow, with the added problems of the coronavirus disease 2019 pandemic making clinical trials difficult to conduct. Even though the utility of combined catheters has already been confirmed in ex vivo examinations, evidence from clinical practice is lacking. The advantage of the combined catheter versus a single imaging modality is clear, however, there are some concerns about using them in lesions with severe tortuosity and severe calcification due to their inferior derivability compared with the latest imaging devices. However, the future combined catheter will have the same deliverability as the single-modality catheters that exist today.

SUMMARY

The combined IVUS-OCT catheter concept is becoming an increasingly attractive option for use in both simple and complex PCI when it can allow the operator to pragmatically choose IVUS/OCT alone or hybrid IVUS-OCT based on clinical needs, while allowing more comprehensive evaluation of plaque composition.

CLINICS CARE POINTS

- The clinical applications of intravascular imaging are (1) a research tool for investigating the progression and regression of CAD with or without drug interventions, (2) qualitative and quantitative assessment of vulnerable plaque, and (3) guiding the indication for PCI and guiding the PCI procedure including sizing of devices, and optimization of the treated lesion.

- The combined IVUS-OCT catheter concept is becoming an increasingly attractive option for use in both simple and complex PCI when it can allow the operator to pragmatically choose IVUS/OCT alone or hybrid IVUS-OCT based on clinical needs while allowing more comprehensive evaluation of plaque composition.

FUNDING

None.

DISCLOSURES

Dr P.W. Serruys reports institutional grants from Sinomedical Sciences Technology, SMT (Sahajanand Medical technological), India, Philips/Volcano, Netherlands, Xeltis, and HeartFlow, outside the submitted work. Dr K. Ninomiya reports a grant from Abbott Medical Japan outside the submitted work. Dr S. Masuda reports a grant from Terumo (Japan) outside the submitted work. Mr I. Mori is an employee of Terumo Corporation. Dr B. Courtney has the following conflicts with Conavi Medical Inc: Shareholder, employment, director, patent royalties, research funding. All other authors have no conflict of interest to declare.

SUPPLEMENTARY DATA

Supplementary data related to this article can be found online at https://doi.org/10.1016/j.iccl.2022.12.002.

REFERENCES

1. Yock PG, Linker DT, Angelsen BA. Two-dimensional intravascular ultrasound: technical development and initial clinical experience. J Am Soc Echocardiogr 1989;2(4):296–304.
2. Brezinski ME, Tearney GJ, Bouma BE, et al. Imaging of coronary artery microstructure (in vitro) with optical coherence tomography. Am J Cardiol 1996;77(1):92–3.
3. Huang D, Swanson EA, Lin CP, et al. Optical coherence tomography. Science 1991;254(5035):1178–81.
4. Jang IK, Bouma BE, Kang DH, et al. Visualization of coronary atherosclerotic plaques in patients using optical coherence tomography: comparison with intravascular ultrasound. J Am Coll Cardiol 2002;39(4):604–9.
5. Bajaj R, Garcia-Garcia HM, Courtney BK, et al. Multi-modality intravascular imaging for guiding coronary intervention and assessing coronary atheroma: the Novasight Hybrid IVUS-OCT system. Minerva Cardiol Angiol 2021;69(6):655–70.
6. Ali ZA, Karimi Galougahi K, Mintz GS, et al. Intracoronary optical coherence tomography: state of the art and future directions. EuroIntervention 2021;17(2):e105–23.
7. Ali ZA, Maehara A, Genereux P, et al. Optical coherence tomography compared with intravascular ultrasound and with angiography to guide coronary stent implantation (ILUMIEN III:

OPTIMIZE PCI): a randomised controlled trial. Lancet 2016;388(10060):2618–28.

8. Choi SY, Witzenbichler B, Maehara A, et al. Intravascular ultrasound findings of early stent thrombosis after primary percutaneous intervention in acute myocardial infarction: a Harmonizing Outcomes with Revascularization and Stents in Acute Myocardial Infarction (HORIZONS-AMI) substudy. Circ Cardiovasc Interv 2011;4(3):239–47.

9. Adriaenssens T, Joner M, Godschalk TC, et al. Optical Coherence Tomography Findings in Patients With Coronary Stent Thrombosis: a Report of the PRESTIGE Consortium (Prevention of Late Stent Thrombosis by an Interdisciplinary Global European Effort). Circulation 2017;136(11):1007–21.

10. Radu MD, Raber L, Kalesan B, et al. Coronary evaginations are associated with positive vessel remodelling and are nearly absent following implantation of newer-generation drug-eluting stents: an optical coherence tomography and intravascular ultrasound study. Eur Heart J 2014;35(12):795–807.

11. Sakakura K, Yamamoto K, Taniguchi Y, et al. Intravascular ultrasound enhances the safety of rotational atherectomy. Cardiovasc Revasc Med 2018; 19(3 Pt A):286–91.

12. Zeng Y, Cavalcante R, Collet C, et al. Coronary calcification as a mechanism of plaque/media shrinkage in vessels treated with bioresorbable vascular scaffold: A multimodality intracoronary imaging study. Atherosclerosis 2018;269:6–13.

13. Escaned J, Baptista J, Di Mario C, et al. Significance of automated stenosis detection during quantitative angiography. Insights gained from intracoronary ultrasound imaging. Circulation 1996;94(5):966–72.

14. Serruys PW, Foley DP. Feyter PJd. Quantitative coronary angiograpghy in clinical practice. Developments in Cardiovascular. Medicine 1994.

15. Park SJ, Ahn JM, Kang SJ, et al. Intravascular ultrasound-derived minimal lumen area criteria for functionally significant left main coronary artery stenosis. JACC Cardiovasc Interv 2014;7(8):868–74.

16. Nair A, Margolis MP, Kuban BD, et al. Automated coronary plaque characterisation with intravascular ultrasound backscatter: ex vivo validation. EuroIntervention 2007;3(1):113–20.

17. Jang IK, Tearney GJ, MacNeill B, et al. In vivo characterization of coronary atherosclerotic plaque by use of optical coherence tomography. Circulation 2005;111(12):1551–5.

18. Neumann FJ, Sousa-Uva M, Ahlsson A, et al. 2018 ESC/EACTS Guidelines on myocardial revascularization. Eur Heart J 2019;40(2):87–165.

19. Lawton JS, Tamis-Holland JE, Bangalore S, et al. 2021 ACC/AHA/SCAI Guideline for Coronary Artery Revascularization: Executive Summary: A Report of the American College of Cardiology/ American Heart Association Joint Committee on Clinical Practice Guidelines. Circulation 2022; 145(3):e4–17.

20. Nakamura M, Yaku H, Ako J, et al. JCS/JSCVS 2018 Guideline on Revascularization of Stable Coronary Artery Disease. Circ J 2022;86(3):477–588.

21. Rieber J, Meissner O, Babaryka G, et al. Diagnostic accuracy of optical coherence tomography and intravascular ultrasound for the detection and characterization of atherosclerotic plaque composition in ex-vivo coronary specimens: a comparison with histology. Coron Artery Dis 2006;17(5):425–30.

22. Li J, Li X, Mohar D, et al. Integrated IVUS-OCT for real-time imaging of coronary atherosclerosis. JACC Cardiovasc Imaging 2014;7(1):101–3.

23. Raber L, Heo JH, Radu MD, et al. Offline fusion of co-registered intravascular ultrasound and frequency domain optical coherence tomography images for the analysis of human atherosclerotic plaques. EuroIntervention 2012;8(1):98–108.

24. Sheth TN, Pinilla-Echeverri N, Mehta SR, et al. First-in-Human Images of Coronary Atherosclerosis and Coronary Stents Using a Novel Hybrid Intravascular Ultrasound and Optical Coherence Tomographic Catheter. JACC Cardiovasc Interv 2018;11(23):2427–30.

25. Li X, Yin J, Hu C, et al. High-resolution coregistered intravascular imaging with integrated ultrasound and optical coherence tomography probe. Appl Phys Lett 2010;97(13):133702.

26. Yang HC, Yin J, Hu C, et al. A dual-modality probe utilizing intravascular ultrasound and optical coherence tomography for intravascular imaging applications. IEEE Trans Ultrason Ferroelectr Freq Control 2010;57(12):2839–43.

27. Yin J, Yang HC, Li X, et al. Integrated intravascular optical coherence tomography ultrasound imaging system. J Biomed Opt 2010;15(1):010512.

28. Yin J, Li X, Jing J, et al. Novel combined miniature optical coherence tomography ultrasound probe for in vivo intravascular imaging. J Biomed Opt 2011;16(6):060505.

29. Li BH, Leung AS, Soong A, et al. Hybrid intravascular ultrasound and optical coherence tomography catheter for imaging of coronary atherosclerosis. Catheter Cardiovasc Interv 2013; 81(3):494–507.

30. Li J, Ma T, Jing J, et al. Miniature optical coherence tomography-ultrasound probe for automatically coregistered three-dimensional intracoronary imaging with real-time display. J Biomed Opt 2013; 18(10):100502.

31. Li J, Ma T, Mohar D, et al. Ultrafast optical-ultrasonic system and miniaturized catheter for imaging and characterizing atherosclerotic plaques in vivo. Sci Rep 2015;5:18406.

32. Okamura T, Onuma Y, Garcia-Garcia HM, et al. First-in-man evaluation of intravascular optical

frequency domain imaging (OFDI) of Terumo: a comparison with intravascular ultrasound and quantitative coronary angiography. EuroIntervention 2011;6(9):1037–45.

33. Ono M, Kawashima H, Hara H, et al. Advances in IVUS/OCT and Future Clinical Perspective of Novel Hybrid Catheter System in Coronary Imaging. Front Cardiovasc Med 2020;7:119.

34. Available at: https://panovision-med.com/hxcp Accessed January 27, 2023.

35. Sheth TN, Pinilla-Echeverri N, Mehta SR, et al. First-in-Human Images of Coronary Atherosclerosis and Coronary Stents Using a Novel Hybrid Intravascular Ultrasound and Optical Coherence Tomographic Catheter. JACC Cardiovasc Interv 2018;11(23):2427–30.

36. Gragnano F, Calabro P. Role of dual lipid-lowering therapy in coronary atherosclerosis regression: Evidence from recent studies. Atherosclerosis 2018;269:219–28.

37. Gogas BD, Farooq V, Serruys PW, et al. Assessment of coronary atherosclerosis by IVUS and IVUS-based imaging modalities: progression and regression studies, tissue composition and beyond. Int J Cardiovasc Imaging 2011;27(2):225–37.

38. Puri R, Nissen SE, Ballantyne CM, et al. Factors underlying regression of coronary atheroma with potent statin therapy. Eur Heart J 2013;34(24):1818–25.

39. Kataoka Y, Wolski K, Balog C, et al. Progression of coronary atherosclerosis in stable patients with ultrasonic features of high-risk plaques. Eur Heart J Cardiovasc Imaging 2014;15(9):1035–41.

40. Nicholls SJ, Puri R, Anderson T, et al. Effect of Evolocumab on Progression of Coronary Disease in Statin-Treated Patients: The GLAGOV Randomized Clinical Trial. JAMA 2016;316(22):2373–84.

41. Nishiguchi T, Kubo T, Tanimoto T, et al. Effect of Early Pitavastatin Therapy on Coronary Fibrous-Cap Thickness Assessed by Optical Coherence Tomography in Patients With Acute Coronary Syndrome: The ESCORT Study. JACC Cardiovasc Imaging 2018;11(6):829–38.

42. Raber L, Ueki Y, Otsuka T, et al. Effect of Alirocumab Added to High-Intensity Statin Therapy on Coronary Atherosclerosis in Patients With Acute Myocardial Infarction: The PACMAN-AMI Randomized Clinical Trial. JAMA 2022;327(18):1771–81.

43. Engelen SE, Robinson AJB, Zurke YX, et al. Therapeutic strategies targeting inflammation and immunity in atherosclerosis: how to proceed? Nat Rev Cardiol 2022;19(8):522–42.

44. Ridker PM, Everett BM, Thuren T, et al. Antiinflammatory Therapy with Canakinumab for Atherosclerotic Disease. N Engl J Med 2017;377(12):1119–31.

45. Tardif JC, Kouz S, Waters DD, et al. Efficacy and Safety of Low-Dose Colchicine after Myocardial Infarction. N Engl J Med 2019;381(26):2497–505.

46. Nidorf SM, Fiolet ATL, Mosterd A, et al. Colchicine in Patients with Chronic Coronary Disease. N Engl J Med 2020;383(19):1838–47.

47. Muller JE, Tofler GH, Stone PH. Circadian variation and triggers of onset of acute cardiovascular disease. Circulation 1989;79(4):733–43.

48. Naghavi M, Libby P, Falk E, et al. From vulnerable plaque to vulnerable patient: a call for new definitions and risk assessment strategies: Part I. Circulation 2003;108(14):1664–72.

49. Naghavi M, Libby P, Falk E, et al. From vulnerable plaque to vulnerable patient: a call for new definitions and risk assessment strategies: Part II. Circulation 2003;108(15):1772–8.

50. Stone GW, Maehara A, Lansky AJ, et al. A prospective natural-history study of coronary atherosclerosis. N Engl J Med 2011;364(3):226–35.

51. Raber L, Taniwaki M, Zaugg S, et al. Effect of high-intensity statin therapy on atherosclerosis in non-infarct-related coronary arteries (IBIS-4): a serial intravascular ultrasonography study. Eur Heart J 2015;36(8):490–500.

52. Waksman R, Di Mario C, Torguson R, et al. Identification of patients and plaques vulnerable to future coronary events with near-infrared spectroscopy intravascular ultrasound imaging: a prospective, cohort study. Lancet 2019;394(10209):1629–37.

53. Erlinge D, Maehara A, Ben-Yehuda O, et al. Identification of vulnerable plaques and patients by intracoronary near-infrared spectroscopy and ultrasound (PROSPECT II): a prospective natural history study. Lancet 2021;397(10278):985–95.

54. Kedhi E, Berta B, Roleder T, et al. Thin-cap fibroatheroma predicts clinical events in diabetic patients with normal fractional flow reserve: the COMBINE OCT-FFR trial. Eur Heart J 2021;42(45):4671–9.

55. Prati F, Romagnoli E, Gatto L, et al. Relationship between coronary plaque morphology of the left anterior descending artery and 12 months clinical outcome: the CLIMA study. Eur Heart J 2020;41(3):383–91.

56. Hong SJ, Kim BK, Shin DH, et al. Effect of Intravascular Ultrasound-Guided vs Angiography-Guided Everolimus-Eluting Stent Implantation: The IVUS-XPL Randomized Clinical Trial. JAMA 2015;314(20):2155–63.

57. Hong SJ, Mintz GS, Ahn CM, et al. Effect of Intravascular Ultrasound-Guided Drug-Eluting Stent Implantation: 5-Year Follow-Up of the IVUS-XPL Randomized Trial. JACC Cardiovasc Interv 2020;13(1):62–71.

58. Chieffo A, Latib A, Caussin C, et al. A prospective, randomized trial of intravascular-ultrasound guided compared to angiography guided stent implantation in complex coronary lesions: the AVIO trial. Am Heart J 2013;165(1):65–72.

59. Zhang J, Gao X, Kan J, et al. Intravascular Ultrasound Versus Angiography-Guided Drug-Eluting

Stent Implantation: The ULTIMATE Trial. J Am Coll Cardiol 2018;72(24):3126–37.

60. Gao XF, Ge Z, Kong XQ, et al. 3-Year Outcomes of the ULTIMATE Trial Comparing Intravascular Ultrasound Versus Angiography-Guided Drug-Eluting Stent Implantation. JACC Cardiovasc Interv 2021;14(3):247–57.

61. Onuma Y, Kogame N, Sotomi Y, et al. A Randomized Trial Evaluating Online 3-Dimensional Optical Frequency Domain Imaging-Guided Percutaneous Coronary Intervention in Bifurcation Lesions. Circ Cardiovasc Interv 2020; 13(12):e009183.

62. Amabile N, Range G, Souteyrand G, et al. Optical coherence tomography to guide percutaneous coronary intervention of the left main coronary artery: the LEMON study. EuroIntervention 2021;17(2):e124–31.

63. Maehara A, Ben-Yehuda O, Ali Z, et al. Comparison of Stent Expansion Guided by Optical Coherence Tomography Versus Intravascular Ultrasound: The ILUMIEN II Study (Observational Study of Optical Coherence Tomography [OCT] in Patients Undergoing Fractional Flow Reserve [FFR] and Percutaneous Coronary Intervention). JACC Cardiovasc Interv 2015;8(13):1704–14.

64. Kubo T, Shinke T, Okamura T, et al. Optical frequency domain imaging vs. intravascular ultrasound in percutaneous coronary intervention (OPINION trial): one-year angiographic and clinical results. Eur Heart J 2017;38(42):3139–47.

65. Katagiri Y, Tenekecioglu E, Serruys PW, et al. What does the future hold for novel intravascular imaging devices: a focus on morphological and physiological assessment of plaque. Expert Rev Med Devices 2017;14(12):985–99.

66. Kim S, Nam HS, Lee MW, et al. Comprehensive Assessment of High-Risk Plaques by Dual-Modal Imaging Catheter in Coronary Artery. JACC Basic Transl Sci 2021;6(12):948–60.

67. Kuku KO, Singh M, Ozaki Y, et al. Near-Infrared Spectroscopy Intravascular Ultrasound Imaging: State of the Art. Front Cardiovasc Med 2020;7:107.

68. Muller J, Madder R. OCT-NIRS Imaging for Detection of Coronary Plaque Structure and Vulnerability. Front Cardiovasc Med 2020;7:90.

Optical Coherence Tomography in Vulnerable Plaque and Acute Coronary Syndrome

Takashi Kubo, MD

KEYWORDS

- Acute coronary syndrome • Plaque rupture • Plaque erosion • Calcified nodule
- Optical coherence tomography • Thin-cap fibroatheroma • Vulnerable plaque

---

KEY POINTS

- Optical coherence tomography (OCT) can detect plaque rupture, plaque erosion, and calcified nodule in the culprit lesions of acute coronary syndrome.
- OCT can detect vulnerable plaque features such as thin fibrous caps, large lipid cores, macrophages accumulation, intraplaque microvasculature, cholesterol crystals, healed plaques, and intraplaque hemorrhage.
- OCT can identify patients and plaques at high risk for future coronary events.

INTRODUCTION

Optical coherence tomography (OCT) is an intravascular imaging technique that uses near-infrared light. OCT provides high-resolution cross-sectional images of coronary arteries and enables tissue characterization of atherosclerotic plaques.[1] OCT allows us to observe the culprit lesions of acute coronary syndrome (ACS) in vivo. OCT can identify plaque rupture, plaque erosion, and calcified nodule. Importantly, optimal treatment strategies and prognosis are different among these plaque phenotypes determined by OCT in the ACS culprit lesions. In addition, in cases with atypical symptoms or no obstructive coronary lesions on angiography (eg, myocardial infarction [MI] with nonobstructive coronary arteries), OCT helps distinguish between atherosclerotic ACS and non-atherosclerotic acute coronary events (eg, spontaneous coronary artery dissection [SCAD]). Furthermore, OCT can detect important morphologic features of vulnerable plaque such as a thin fibrous cap, large lipid core,

macrophages accumulation, intraplaque microvasculature, cholesterol crystal, healed plaque, and intraplaque hemorrhage. OCT gives us a valuable opportunity to evaluate the pathophysiology of coronary artery disease and the natural course of coronary atherosclerosis in a clinical setting.

TISSUE CHARACTERIZATION

Histologic validation studies established OCT definitions for key tissues of coronary artery walls and atherosclerotic plaques.[2] Intima is characterized as a signal-rich inner layer; media as a signal-poor middle layer; and adventitia as a signal-rich outer layer (Fig. 1A). Fibrous plaque is defined by a homogeneous, signal-rich region (Fig. 1B). Calcium is defined by a well-delineated, signal-poor region with sharp border (Fig. 1C). Lipid is defined by a signal-poor region with diffuse border (Fig. 1D). Thrombus is defined by a mass protruding into the lumen with signal attenuation. Red blood cell-rich thrombus (called red thrombus) is highly

---

Department of Cardiovascular Medicine, Naga Municipal Hospital, 1282 Uchita, Kinokawa, Wakayama 649-6414, Japan

E-mail address: takakubo@wakayama-med.ac.jp

Intervent Cardiol Clin 12 (2023) 203–214
https://doi.org/10.1016/j.iccl.2022.10.005
2211-7458/23/© 2022 Elsevier Inc. All rights reserved.

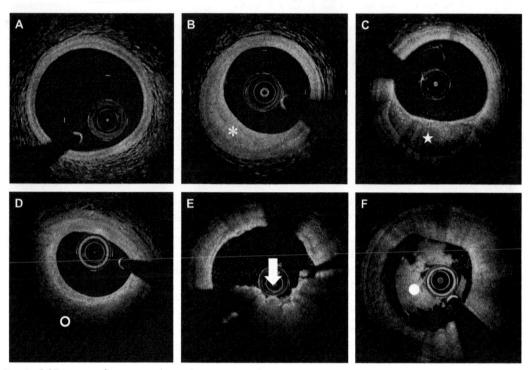

Fig. 1. OCT images of coronary atherosclerosis. Normal coronary artery (*A*). Fibrous plaque (*asterisk*) (*B*). Calcified plaque (*star*) (*C*). Lipidic plaque (*open circle*) (*D*). Red thrombus (*arrow*) (*E*). White thrombus (*closed circle*) (*F*). OCT, optical coherence tomography.

backscattering and has a high attenuation (Fig. 1E). Platelet-rich thrombus (called white thrombus) is less backscattering, is homogeneous, and has low attenuation (Fig. 1F). These OCT definitions were highly sensitive (ranging from 71% to 96%) and specific (ranging from 90% to 98%) for characterizing atherosclerotic plaques and formed the basis for the interpretation of OCT images.[3] Nowadays, OCT software using artificial intelligence allows automated tissue characterization with excellent diagnostic accuracy (98% [95% confidence interval {CI}: 93%–99%] in fibrous plaque, 89% [95%CI: 82%–93%] in calcium, and 91% [95%CI: 85%–94%] in lipid).[4]

ACUTE CORONARY SYNDROME CULPRIT LESIONS

Plaque Rupture

Plaque rupture is found by OCT in ≈40% of the culprit lesions of ACS (Fig. 2A). Plaque rupture is defined by the presence of fibrous cap discontinuity with a clear cavity formed inside the plaque. The ACS culprit lesions with plaque rupture often have a thin fibrous cap, large lipidic plaque, macrophages accumulation, cholesterol crystals, and spotty calcium deposits (defined by a calcium arc <90°).[5] The disrupted

fibrous cap is thinner in the culprit plaques of rest-onset ACS compared with exertion-triggered ACS.[6] The cavity inside the plaque is larger in ST-segment elevation MI (STEMI) than non-ST-segment elevation ACS (NSTEACS).[7] Plaque rupture often has abundant thrombi, which may cause artery-to-artery embolic MI due to the migration of thrombus formed at the proximal segment of the culprit coronary artery.[8] Plaque rupture in the ACS culprit lesion is associated with poor percutaneous coronary intervention (PCI) results (such as slow flow, no-reflow, distal embolism, and irregular tissue protrusion after stent implantation) and worse long-term clinical outcomes.[9] In addition, the patients with ACS caused by plaque rupture have an increased risk of subsequent acute coronary events arising from non-culprit lesions. The patients with ACS caused by plaque rupture exhibit multiple thin-capped fibroatheromas (TCFAs) and severe vascular inflammation in three coronary arteries.[10] The fibrous cap of the non-culprit lesions becomes even thinner in the weeks following the onset of ACS.[11]

Plaque Erosion

Plaque erosion is found by OCT in ≈30% of the culprit lesions of ACS (Fig. 2B). Plaque erosion is

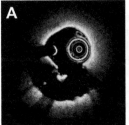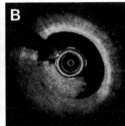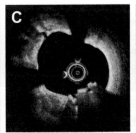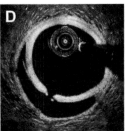

Fig. 2. OCT images of ACS culprit lesions. Plaque rupture (A). Plaque erosion (B). Calcified nodule (C). Spontaneous coronary artery dissection (D). ACS, acute coronary syndrome. OCT, optical coherence tomography.

defined by the presence of attached thrombus overlying an intact and visualized plaque, luminal surface irregularity at the culprit lesion in the absence of thrombus, or attenuation of underlying plaque by thrombus without superficial lipid or calcification immediately proximal or distal to the site of thrombus.[12] The OCT metric of plaque erosion is different from the pathologic definition, and therefore, the term "OCT-erosion" or "intact fibrous cap" may be used instead of erosion. Plaque erosion has different clinical characteristics when compared with plaque rupture. Patients with plaque erosion are more likely to be young, female, and smokers.[12] Plaque erosion is more often identified in the culprit lesions of NSTEACS than STEMI and may be found in coronary arteries responsible for vasospastic angina.[13] The ACS culprit lesions with plaque erosion often show eccentric fibrotic plaques, small plaque burden, and negative vessel remodeling when assessed by intravascular ultrasound (IVUS).[14] In addition, the ACS culprit lesions with plaque erosion show a smaller value of lipid core burden index in near-infrared spectroscopy (NIRS) and have a lower frequency of low-density (defined as <30 HU) plaques in coronary computed tomography angiography (CTA) compared with those with plaque rupture.[15–17]

Acute results of PCI are better in plaque erosion than in plaque rupture. Plaque erosion has a lower frequency of incomplete stent apposition, thrombus or tissue protrusion, slow flow, no-reflow, and distal embolism.[14] Acute myocardial infarction (AMI) caused by plaque erosion shows a lower serum creatine kinase elevation, smaller transmural MI extent, less microvascular obstruction, and higher left ventricular ejection fraction.[18]

Long-term prognosis after PCI is also better in plaque erosion than in plaque rupture. Niccoli and colleagues showed that the frequency of major adverse cardiovascular event (MACE) (defined as a composite of cardiac death and nonfatal MI) during a 32-month follow-up after PCI was significantly lower in plaque erosion than in plaque rupture (39% vs 14%, $P = .001$).[19] Yonetsu and colleagues demonstrated that the frequency of MACE (defined as a composite of death, MI, revascularization, and congestive heart failure requiring hospitalization) during a 21-month follow-up after PCI was significantly lower in plaque erosion than in plaque rupture (36% vs 22%, $P = .012$).[20]

A couple of studies showed that patients with ACS caused by plaque erosion might be stabilized by antithrombotic therapy without stent implantation. Prati and colleagues showed that 12 patients with STEMI caused by plaque erosion were treated with thrombus aspiration and dual-antiplatelet therapy without stenting, and no patient had MACE (defined as a composite of death, MI, target lesion revascularization [TLR], or heart failure) during a 2-year follow-up.[21] Hu and colleagues demonstrated that 13 patients with ACS caused by plaque erosion managed with conservative treatment without stenting had no MACE (defined as a composite of death, nonfatal MI, or revascularization) during a 1-year follow-up.[22] Jia and colleagues conducted a single-center prospective study named EROSION to investigate the feasibility of the conservative treatment without stenting in 60 patients with ACS caused by plaque erosion.[23,24] When plaque erosion was diagnosed by OCT, the angiographic diameter stenosis in the culprit lesion was less than 70%, thrombolysis in MI flow grade was 3, and the patient had no chest symptoms. Without receiving stent implantation, the patients were continuously treated with aspirin (300 mg loading dose and 100 mg daily thereafter) and ticagrelor (180 mg loading dose and 90 mg twice per day thereafter). At 1-month follow-up, 78% of the patients had greater than 50% reduction of thrombus volume compared with baseline, and 37% of the patients had no visible thrombus as assessed by OCT. At 12-month follow-up, 93% of the patients were free of MACE (defined as a composite of cardiac death, recurrent MI, ischemia-driven TLR, stroke, and major bleeding), although 6% of the patients required revascularization due to exertional angina and 2% of the patients had gastrointestinal bleeding.

Calcified Nodule

Calcified nodule is found by OCT in ≈10% of the culprit lesions of ACS (Fig. 2C). Calcified nodule is defined by a fibrous cap disruption detected over a calcified plaque characterized by protruding calcification, superficial calcium, or the presence of substantive calcium proximal and/or distal to the lesion.[12] Calcified nodule is common in ACS patients of elderly, female, diabetes mellitus, and chronic renal failure treated with hemodialysis.[25] Calcified nodule is often located in ostial and mid right coronary artery (RCA) and is associated with severe calcification and large hinge movement of the vessel.[26] More than 50% of the ACS culprit lesions with calcified nodule show negative remodeling.[14] Calcified nodule is associated with an increased risk of stent underexpansion.[27] The effectiveness of rotablator atherectomy, orbital atherectomy, directional coronary atherectomy, excimer laser catheter ablation, and intravascular lithotripsy for calcified nodule remains controversial.[28] The long-term prognosis of PCI for calcified nodule has not yet been fully elucidated. Recent studies have reported that calcified nodules can protrude through the stent struts early after PCI and cause stent thrombosis and restenosis.[29,30]

Spontaneous Coronary Artery Dissection

SCAD is one cause of non-atherosclerotic ACS and is found by OCT in up to 4% of ACS (Fig. 2D).[31] In angiographically suspected SCAD with obstructive but normal coronary flow, the use of OCT is recommended for diagnostic and therapeutic guidance.[32] OCT can identify true and false lumen, intimal flaps, entries, reentries, and hematomas. The OCT imaging procedure with contrast injection results in a slight but a significant increase in intracoronary pressure (9 ± 2 mm Hg in systole).[33] It is necessary to understand the risk of extension of SCAD due to the OCT imaging procedure.

VULNERABLE PLAQUE
Morphologic Features

OCT can detect morphologic features of vulnerable plaques. OCT can identify TCFA with a minimum fibrous cap thickness of less than 65 μm, which is a potential precursor lesion of plaque rupture (Fig. 3A). Histologic validation studies showed that OCT can accurately measure the thickness of the fibrous cap above the lipid core.[34] Lipid size is estimated by measuring the angle of the lipid (called lipid arc) in a cross-section. Lipid-rich plaque (LRP) is defined by a maximum lipid arc of greater than 90° (or >180°). TCFA and LRP determined by OCT are well associated with attenuated plaques by IVUS, intensive yellow plaques by angioscopy, low-density plaques by coronary CTA, and moderately associated with TCFAs by virtual histology IVUS and large lipid core burden index by NIRS. A three-vessel OCT study in patients with ACS showed that non-culprit TCFA was most frequently found in the proximal left anterior descending artery (LAD) followed by the proximal and mid RCA and the proximal left circumflex artery.[35]

OCT allows further identification of several microstructures of vulnerable plaques previously only observable in pathology. Macrophages accumulation is identified as a signal-rich, distinct, or confluent punctate region with rapid signal attenuation (Fig. 3B). Macrophages accumulation is often seen at the boundary between the bottom of the fibrous cap and the top of a lipid core. The ACS patients caused by plaque rupture frequently have a high macrophage density not only in culprit lesions but also in non-culprit lesions.[36]

Intraplaque microvasculature (ie, vasa vasorum) is identified as a low-intensity luminal structure within the plaque and can usually be followed in multiple contiguous frames (Fig. 3C). Intraplaque microvasculature volume is associated with plaque burden.[37]

Cholesterol crystals are identified as thin, linear, high-intensity regions without significant signal attenuation (Fig. 3D). A histologic validation study showed that OCT had a sensitivity of 68% and specificity of 92% for the detection of cholesterol crystals.[38] Cholesterol crystals are often detected in the ACS culprit lesions with plaque rupture and are associated with a thin fibrous cap and a large lipid arc.[39]

Healed plaques, which are formed due to recurrent silent plaque rupture and subsequent healing or silent plaque erosion and thrombosis, are identified as layered plaques by OCT (Fig. 3E). Healed plaques are defined by OCT as a heterogeneous signal-rich layer of different optical intensity located close to the luminal surface with clear demarcation from the underlying plaque. A histologic validation study showed that OCT had a sensitivity of 81% and specificity of 98% for the detection of healed plaques.[40] Healed plaques are associated with small

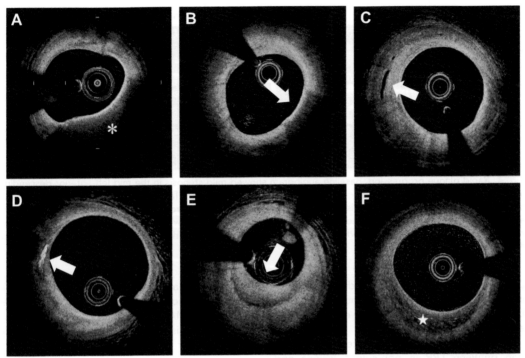

Fig. 3. OCT images of vulnerable plaque features. Thin-cap fibroatheroma (*asterisk*) (*A*). Macrophages accumulation (*arrow*) (*B*). Intraplaque microvasculature (*arrow*) (*C*). Cholesterol crystal (*arrow*) (*D*). Healed plaque (*arrow*) (*E*). Intraplaque hemorrhage (*star*) (*F*). OCT, optical coherence tomography.

minimal lumen area, thin fibrous cap, and presence of LRP, macrophages accumulation, intraplaque microvasculature, and spotty calcium deposits.[41] Recent studies showed that ACS patients with a layered plaque at the culprit lesion had higher cardiovascular risk profiles, elevated biomarkers of systemic inflammation, more multivessel disease, higher angiographic complexity of the culprit/non-culprit lesions, and a higher MACE rate.[42–45]

Intraplaque hemorrhage is identified as a homogeneous low-intensity region without attenuation (Fig. 3F). Intraplaque hemorrhage has a various appearance depending on time from the hemorrhagic event and may be hidden in an advanced necrotic core because of signal attenuation. Intraplaque hemorrhage is frequently colocated with cholesterol crystals (82% at the lesion level).[46] Intraplaque hemorrhage may contribute to rapid plaque progression, luminal narrowing, and plaque destabilization.

Prediction of Plaque Progression

OCT can predict the progression of coronary artery lesions (Fig. 4). To date, four studies have investigated the association between baseline OCT findings and subsequent progression of coronary lesions as assessed by serial (baseline and follow-up) angiography or IVUS. Uemura and colleagues showed that TCFA and intraplaque microvasculature were associated with subsequent rapid lesion progression defined as a decrease of angiographic minimum lumen diameter greater than 0.4 mm at 7-month follow-up.[47] Araki and colleagues demonstrated that LRP, TCFA, and layered plaques were predictors of angiographic lesion progression (defined as above) at 7-month follow-up.[48] Yamamoto and colleagues showed that lipid plaques often developed into healed plaques during 8-month follow-up, leading to the lesion progression defined as a decrease of an IVUS lumen area greater than 0.5 mm^2.[49] Xie and colleagues demonstrated that TCFA and intraplaque microvasculature were associated with plaque progression defined as an increase of IVUS plaque volume $\geq$5% at 12-month follow-up[50]

Identification of Vulnerable Patient

OCT can identify vulnerable patients by assessing non-culprit lesions in coronary arteries. Based on patient-level analysis, two studies evaluated the association between the baseline OCT characteristics of non-culprit lesions and follow-

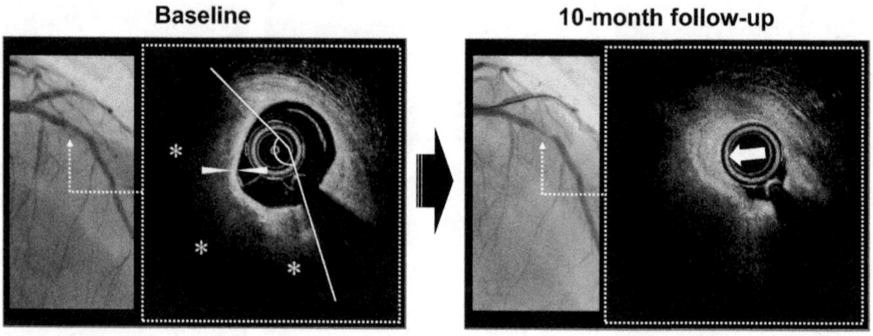

Baseline   **10-month follow-up**

Fig. 4. Rapid plaque progression. Baseline angiogram showed mild stenosis in the mid left anterior descending artery. Baseline OCT identified an LRP (maximum lipid arc = 150° [asterisks] and minimum fibrous cap thickness = 100 μm [arrowheads]). This plaque was associated with lesion progression 10 months after baseline imaging. Follow-up angiography showed severe stenosis in the lesion. Follow-up OCT detected healed plaque (arrow) in the lesion that was imaged during baseline OCT. LRP, lipid-rich plaque; OCT, optical coherence tomography.

up MACE. These studies included MACE resulting from non-culprit lesions not assessed by baseline OCT as well as non-culprit lesions assessed by baseline OCT.

Xing and colleagues investigated the association between LRP in non-culprit lesions and follow-up MACE in 1474 patients in the international, multicenter OCT registry by Massachusetts General Hospital, Boston, USA.[51] The non-culprit LRP was defined as a lipid plaque that was not related to the index event and had lipid arc of greater than 90° by OCT. MACE was defined as a composite of cardiac death, MI, and ischemia-driven revascularization. The frequency of MACE during a 2-year follow-up was significantly higher in patients with LRP than in those without LRP (7.2% vs 2.6%, P = .033). Longer lipid length (lipid length >5.9 mm), larger lipid arc (maximum lipid arc >192.8°), and more severe stenosis (percent area stenosis >68.5%) were independent predictors of MACE.

Prati and colleagues investigated the association between non-culprit plaque morphology in proximal LAD and clinical outcomes in 1003 patients in the prospective, multicenter OCT registry named CLIMA.[52] The presence of a combination of minimum lumen area less than 3.5 mm^2, fibrous cap thickness less than 75 μm, lipid arc greater than 180°, and macrophages accumulation was assessed by OCT in the non-culprit lesions of proximal LAD. MACE was defined as a composite of cardiac death or MI. The frequency of MACE during a 1-year follow-up was significantly higher in patients with these four prespecified plaque features than in those without (19.4% vs 3.1%, hazard ratio [HR] 7.54 [95%CI: 3.1–18.6], P < .001). The presence of

these four plaque features showed low sensitivity (19%) and high specificity (98%) for the prediction of MACE. Thereafter, the post hoc analysis of this registry added calcified nodule as a predictor of MACE.[53,54]

Identification of Vulnerable Plaque

OCT may be able to identify vulnerable plaques (Figs. 5–8). Based on lesion-level analysis, four studies evaluated the association between baseline OCT characteristics of non-culprit lesions and follow-up MACE resulting from the non-culprit lesions observed by baseline OCT (ie, lesion-specific MACE).

Kubo and colleagues investigated the association between lipidic plaques characterized as both LRP (defined by maximum lipid arc >180°) and TCFA versus lesion-specific follow-up ACS events in 3533 non-culprit lesions of 1378 patients in the OCT registry at Wakayama Medical University, Wakayama, Japan.[55] The follow-up ACS event was defined as a composite of cardiac death, MI, and unstable angina with coronary thrombosis determined by follow-up OCT. The frequency of the ACS events during a 7-year follow-up was significantly higher in lipidic plaques that were characterized as both LRP and TCFA than lipidic plaques that did not have these characteristics (33% vs 2%, HR 19.14 [95%CI: 11.74–31.20], P < .001). The presence of both LRP and TCFA showed low sensitivity (38%) and high specificity (97%) for predicting the follow-up ACS events. The maximum lipid arc greater than 185°, minimum fibrous cap thickness less than 150 μm, and minimum lumen area less than 2.90 mm^2 were independent predictors of the follow-up ACS events.

Baseline   **7-month follow-up**   **25-month follow-up**

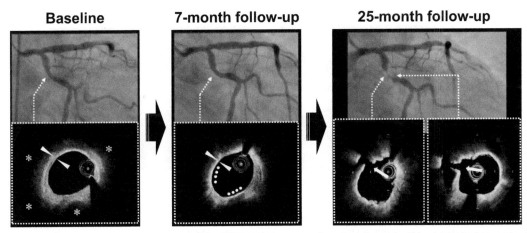

Fig. 5. AMI due to plaque rupture arising from TCFA. Angiogram at baseline showed mild stenosis in the proximal left circumflex artery. OCT at baseline characterized the plaque as LRP (maximum lipid arc = 360° [*asterisks*] and minimum fibrous cap thickness = 140 μm [*arrowheads*]). Angiogram at 7-month follow-up showed no progression in the stenosis. OCT at 7-month follow-up showed the decrease of the fibrous cap thickness and the presence of macrophages accumulation (*dots*), characterizing this plaque as both LRP and TCFA (minimum fibrous cap thickness = 60 μm [*arrowheads*]). This plaque was associated with myocardial infarction 25 months after baseline imaging. Angiography at 25-month follow-up showed that the stenosis developed into a subtotal occlusion. OCT at 25-month follow-up showed rupture (*arrows*) of the plaque that was imaged during OCT at baseline and 7-month follow-up. ACS = acute coronary syndrome, LRP, lipid-rich plaque; OCT, optical coherence tomography; TCFA, thin-cap fibroatheroma.

Kedhi and colleagues performed a prospective international natural history study named COMBINE OCT-FFR to investigate the association between TCFA and MACE in 550 nonischemic fractional flow reserve (FFR) (>0.80) lesions in 550 diabetic patients.[56] MACE was defined as a composite of cardiac death, MI, clinically driven TLR, and hospitalization due to unstable or progressive angina. The frequency of MACE during an 18-month follow-up was significantly higher in TCFA than in non-TCFA (13.3% vs 3.1%, HR 4.65 [95%CI: 1.99–10.89], P < .001). The MACE arising from TCFA was mainly driven by MI, which occurred only in TCFA, and clinically driven TLR, which occurred eight times more often in TCFA compared with non-TCFA.

Usui and colleagues investigated the association between healed plaque and MACE in 726 non-culprit lesions of 538 patients in the OCT registry at Tsuchiura Kyodo General Hospital, Ibaraki, Japan.[41] MACE was defined as a composite of cardiac death, MI, and ischemia-

Baseline   **8-month follow-up**

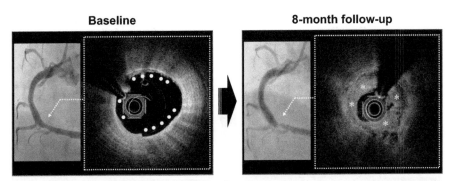

Fig. 6. AMI due to plaque erosion from fibrous plaque. Baseline angiogram showed mild stenosis in the mid right coronary artery. Baseline OCT identified a fibrous plaque with macrophages accumulation (*dots*). This plaque was associated with myocardial infarction 8 months after baseline imaging. Follow-up angiography showed that the stenosis developed into a subtotal occlusion. Follow-up OCT detected thrombus (*asterisks*) overlying intact fibrous cap of the plaque (ie, OCT-erosion) that was imaged during baseline OCT. ACS, acute coronary syndrome; OCT, optical coherence tomography.

Baseline   **9-month follow-up**

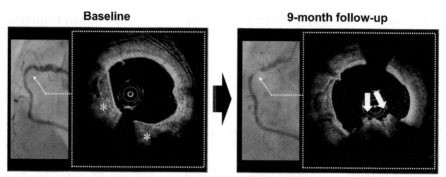

Fig. 7. AMI due to calcified nodule from fibrocalcific plaque. Baseline angiogram showed mild stenosis in the proximal right coronary artery. Baseline OCT identified a plaque with superficial calcium sheet (*asterisks*). This plaque was associated with myocardial infarction 9 months after baseline imaging. Follow-up angiography showed that the stenosis developed into a subtotal occlusion. Follow-up OCT detected calcified nodule (*arrows*) in the plaque that was imaged during baseline OCT. AMI, acute myocardial infarction; OCT, optical coherence tomography.

driven revascularization. The frequency of MACE during a 2-year follow-up was significantly higher in healed plaque than in non-healed plaque (3.7% vs 1.7%, HR 2.01 [95%CI: 1.20–3.37], $P < .01$).

Recently, Usui and colleagues expanded this study and investigated the association between plaques that had both intraplaque hemorrhage and cholesterol crystal versus MACE in 735 non-culprit lesions of 566 patients.[46] The frequency of MACE during a 3-year follow-up was significantly higher in plaques that had both intraplaque hemorrhage and cholesterol crystal than plaques that did not have these characteristics (8.6% vs 1.9%, adjusted HR 3.09 [95%CI: 1.27–7.50], $P = .01$). The presence of both intraplaque hemorrhage and cholesterol crystal showed low sensitivity (45%) and high specificity (85%) for the prediction of MACE. TCFA and minimum lumen area less than 3.5 mm^2 were also independent predictors of MACE.

PLAQUE STABILIZATION

OCT allows evaluation of coronary plaque stabilization by lipid-lowering therapy. Several OCT studies showed that the lipid-lowering therapy with statins, proprotein convertase subtilisin/kexin type 9 (PCSK9) inhibitor, ezetimibe, or eicosapentaenoic acid increased fibrous cap thickness, decreased lipid size, and reduced macrophages accumulation in coronary atherosclerotic plaques.

The EASY-FIT study evaluated the effect of statin therapy on the fibrous cap thickness in coronary plaques using serial OCT at baseline and 1-year follow-up.[57] The increase in fibrous cap was correlated with the decrease in serum atherogenic lipoproteins such as low-density lipoprotein cholesterol (LDL-C) and oxidized LDL and inflammatory biomarkers such as high-sensitive C-reactive protein and matrix metalloproteinase-9 (produced by activated

Baseline   **9-year follow-up**

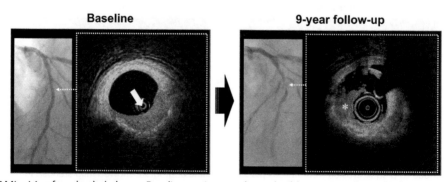

Fig. 8. AMI arising from healed plaque. Baseline angiogram showed mild stenosis in the mid left anterior descending artery. Baseline OCT identified a healed plaque (*arrow*). This plaque was associated with myocardial infarction 9 years after baseline imaging. Follow-up angiography showed that the stenosis developed into a subtotal occlusion. Follow-up OCT detected thrombus (*asterisk*) overlying the plaque that was imaged during baseline OCT. AMI, acute myocardial infarction; OCT, optical coherence tomography.

macrophages and induces collagen breakdown in the fibrous cap) by the statin therapy.

The HUYGENS study assessed the effect of PCSK9 inhibitor in addition to high-intensity statin therapy on plaque phenotype using serial OCT at baseline and 1-year follow-up.[58] The PCSK9 inhibitor group achieved lower LDL-C levels (28.1 vs 87.2 mg/dL, $P < .001$) at 1-year follow-up and showed a greater increase in minimum fibrous cap thickness (+42.7 vs +21.5 μm, $P = .015$) and a greater decrease in maximum lipid arc (−57.5 vs −31.4°, $P = .04$) and macrophage index (−3.17 vs −1.45 mm, $P = .04$) compared with the placebo group.

LIMITATION

OCT has some limitations in observing ACS culprit lesions and vulnerable plaques. First, OCT may not observe coronary arteries with severe stenosis or thrombotic obstruction due to insufficient removal of blood from the lumen by contrast injection. Second, OCT may not observe plaque behind the thrombus due to signal attenuation. Third, OCT has a shallow penetration depth and cannot depict the entire plaque. Therefore, OCT may not estimate plaque burden, which is an important predictor of vulnerable plaque. Finally, OCT may not be used in patients with end-stage renal disease because of the increase of contrast volume for imaging.

FUTURE PERSPECTIVES

Recently, new optical imaging technologies have been developed that enable more detailed evaluation of the pathology of ACS culprit lesions and vulnerable plaques. The hybrid OCT-IVUS system provides the high resolution of OCT with the larger field of view of IVUS.[59] The hybrid OCT-NIRS system provides complementary structural (eg, fibrous cap by OCT) and compositional (ie, lipid by NIRS) data for atherosclerotic plaque.[60] Near-infrared autofluorescence imaging combined with OCT detects fluorescence from naturally occurring molecules and identifies advanced necrotic core-containing lesions and specifically TCFAs.[61] Fluorescence lifetime imaging microscopy combined with OCT measures fluorescence intensity fluctuations and detects regions of high lipid concentration compared with collagen.[62]

SUMMARY

OCT can identify plaque rupture, plaque erosion, and calcified nodule in ACS culprit lesions. OCT also helps find vulnerable patients and vulnerable plaques at high risk for future coronary events. In the clinical setting, OCT provides a better understanding of coronary atherosclerosis and contributes to accurate diagnosis and treatment guidance of coronary artery disease.

CLINICS CARE POINTS

- Plaque rupture is associated with slow flow, no-reflow, distal embolism, and irregular tissue protrusion after stent implantation.

- Plaque erosion has a better clinical outcome after PCI compared with plaque rupture.

- Calcified nodule has an increased risk of stent underexpansion.

- OCT-derived thin fibrous cap and large lipid core in non-culprit plaques are associated with future MACE.

- Intensive lipid-lowering therapy results in increased fibrous cap thickness and decreased lipid arc assessed by OCT.

DISCLOSURE

The author has nothing to disclose.

REFERENCES

1. Tearney GJ, Regar E, Akasaka T, et al. Consensus standards for acquisition, measurement, and reporting of intravascular optical coherence tomography studies: a report from the International Working Group for Intravascular Optical Coherence Tomography Standardization and Validation. J Am Coll Cardiol 2012;59:1058–72.

2. Fujii K, Kubo T, Otake H, et al. Expert consensus statement for quantitative measurement and morphological assessment of optical coherence tomography: update 2022. Cardiovasc Interv Ther 2022;37:248–54.

3. Yabushita H, Bouma BE, Houser SL, et al. Characterization of human atherosclerosis by optical coherence tomography. Circulation 2002;106:1640–5.

4. Chu M, Jia H, Gutiérrez-Chico JL, et al. Artificial intelligence and optical coherence tomography for the automatic characterisation of human atherosclerotic plaques. EuroIntervention 2021;17:41–50.

5. Mizukoshi M, Kubo T, Takarada S, et al. Coronary superficial and spotty calcium deposits in culprit coronary lesions of acute coronary syndrome as

determined by optical coherence tomography. Am J Cardiol 2013;112:34–40.

6. Tanaka A, Imanishi T, Kitabata H, et al. Morphology of exertion-triggered plaque rupture in patients with acute coronary syndrome: an optical coherence tomography study. Circulation 2008;118:2368–73.

7. Ino Y, Kubo T, Tanaka A, et al. Difference of culprit lesion morphologies between ST-segment elevation myocardial infarction and non-ST-segment elevation acute coronary syndrome: an optical coherence tomography study. JACC Cardiovasc Interv 2011;4:76–82.

8. Takahata M, Ino Y, Kubo T, et al. Prevalence, Features, and Prognosis of Artery-to-Artery Embolic ST-Segment-Elevation Myocardial Infarction: An Optical Coherence Tomography Study. J Am Heart Assoc 2020;9:e017661.

9. Soeda T, Uemura S, Park SJ, et al. Incidence and Clinical Significance of Poststent Optical Coherence Tomography Findings: One-Year Follow-Up Study From a Multicenter Registry. Circulation 2015;132:1020–9.

10. Nakajima A, Sugiyama T, Araki M, et al. Plaque Rupture, Compared With Plaque Erosion, Is Associated With a Higher Level of Pancoronary Inflammation. JACC Cardiovasc Imaging 2021. https://doi.org/10.1016/j.jcmg.2021.10.014. S1936-878X(21)00781-00786.

11. Nishiguchi T, Kubo T, Tanimoto T, et al. Effect of Early Pitavastatin Therapy on Coronary Fibrous-Cap Thickness Assessed by Optical Coherence Tomography in Patients With Acute Coronary Syndrome: The ESCORT Study. JACC Cardiovasc Imaging 2018;11:829–38.

12. Jia H, Abtahian F, Aguirre AD, et al. In vivo diagnosis of plaque erosion and calcified nodule in patients with acute coronary syndrome by intravascular optical coherence tomography. J Am Coll Cardiol 2013;62:1748–58.

13. Shin ES, Ann SH, Singh GB, et al. OCT-defined morphological characteristics of coronary artery spasm sites in vasospastic angina. JACC Cardiovasc Imaging 2015;8:1059–67.

14. Higuma T, Soeda T, Abe N, et al. A Combined Optical Coherence Tomography and Intravascular Ultrasound Study on Plaque Rupture, Plaque Erosion, and Calcified Nodule in Patients With ST-Segment Elevation Myocardial Infarction: Incidence, Morphologic Characteristics, and Outcomes After Percutaneous Coronary Intervention. JACC Cardiovasc Interv 2015;8:1166–76.

15. Terada K, Kubo T, Kameyama T, et al. NIRS-IVUS for Differentiating Coronary Plaque Rupture, Erosion, and Calcified Nodule in Acute Myocardial Infarction. JACC Cardiovasc Imaging 2021;14:1440–50.

16. Kubo T, Terada K, Ino Y, et al. Combined Use of Multiple Intravascular Imaging Techniques in Acute Coronary Syndrome. Front Cardiovasc Med 2022;8:824128.

17. Ozaki Y, Okumura M, Ismail TF, et al. Coronary CT angiographic characteristics of culprit lesions in acute coronary syndromes not related to plaque rupture as defined by optical coherence tomography and angioscopy. Eur Heart J 2011;32:2814–23.

18. Satogami K, Ino Y, Kubo T, et al. Impact of Plaque Rupture Detected by Optical Coherence Tomography on Transmural Extent of Infarction After Successful Stenting in ST-Segment Elevation Acute Myocardial Infarction. JACC Cardiovasc Interv 2017;10:1025–33.

19. Niccoli G, Montone RA, Di Vito L, et al. Plaque rupture and intact fibrous cap assessed by optical coherence tomography portend different outcomes in patients with acute coronary syndrome. Eur Heart J 2015;36:1377–84.

20. Yonetsu T, Lee T, Murai T, et al. Plaque morphologies and the clinical prognosis of acute coronary syndrome caused by lesions with intact fibrous cap diagnosed by optical coherence tomography. Int J Cardiol 2016;203:766–74.

21. Prati F, Uemura S, Souteyrand G, et al. OCT-based diagnosis and management of STEMI associated with intact fibrous cap. JACC Cardiovasc Imaging 2013;6:283–7.

22. Hu S, Zhu Y, Zhang Y, et al. Management and Outcome of Patients With Acute Coronary Syndrome Caused by Plaque Rupture Versus Plaque Erosion: An Intravascular Optical Coherence Tomography Study. J Am Heart Assoc 2017;6:e004730.

23. Jia H, Dai J, Hou J, et al. Effective anti-thrombotic therapy without stenting: intravascular optical coherence tomography-based management in plaque erosion (the EROSION study). Eur Heart J 2017;38:792–800.

24. Xing L, Yamamoto E, Sugiyama T, et al. EROSION Study (Effective Anti-Thrombotic Therapy Without Stenting: Intravascular Optical Coherence Tomography-Based Management in Plaque Erosion): A 1-Year Follow-Up Report. Circ Cardiovasc Interv 2017;10:e005860.

25. Ijichi T, Nakazawa G, Torii S, et al. Evaluation of coronary arterial calcification - Ex-vivo assessment by optical frequency domain imaging. Atherosclerosis 2015;243:242–7.

26. Lee T, Mintz GS, Matsumura M, et al. Prevalence, Predictors, and Clinical Presentation of a Calcified Nodule as Assessed by Optical Coherence Tomography. JACC Cardiovasc Imaging 2017;10:883–91.

27. Khalifa AKM, Kubo T, Ino Y, et al. Optical Coherence Tomography Comparison of Percutaneous Coronary Intervention Among Plaque Rupture,

Erosion, and Calcified Nodule in Acute Myocardial Infarction. Circ J 2020;84:911–6.

28. Ashikaga T, Yoshikawa S, Isobe M. The efficacy of excimer laser pretreatment for calcified nodule in acute coronary syndrome. Cardiovasc Revasc Med 2015;16:197–200.

29. Mori H, Finn AV, Atkinson JB, et al. Calcified Nodule: An Early and Late Cause of In-Stent Failure. JACC Cardiovasc Interv 2016;9:e125–6.

30. Nakamura N, Torii S, Tsuchiya H, et al. Formation of Calcified Nodule as a Cause of Early In-Stent Restenosis in Patients Undergoing Dialysis. J Am Heart Assoc 2020;9:e016595.

31. Nishiguchi T, Tanaka A, Ozaki Y, et al. Prevalence of spontaneous coronary artery dissection in patients with acute coronary syndrome. Eur Heart J Acute Cardiovasc Care 2016;5:263–70.

32. Collet JP, Thiele H, Barbato E, et al. 2020 ESC Guidelines for the management of acute coronary syndromes in patients presenting without persistent ST-segment elevation. Eur Heart J 2021;42:1289–367.

33. Shimamura K, Kubo T, Ino Y, et al. Intracoronary pressure increase due to contrast injection for optical coherence tomography imaging. J Cardiol 2020;75:296–301.

34. Kume T, Akasaka T, Kawamoto T, et al. Measurement of the thickness of the fibrous cap by optical coherence tomography. Am Heart J 2006;152:755. e1–4.

35. Araki M, Soeda T, Kim HO, et al. Spatial Distribution of Vulnerable Plaques: Comprehensive In Vivo Coronary Plaque Mapping. JACC Cardiovasc Imaging 2020;13:1989–99.

36. MacNeill BD, Jang IK, Bouma BE, et al. Focal and multi-focal plaque macrophage distributions in patients with acute and stable presentations of coronary artery disease. J Am Coll Cardiol 2004;44:972–9.

37. Taruya A, Tanaka A, Nishiguchi T, et al. Vasa Vasorum Restructuring in Human Atherosclerotic Plaque Vulnerability: A Clinical Optical Coherence Tomography Study. J Am Coll Cardiol 2015;65:2469–77.

38. Katayama Y, Tanaka A, Taruya A, et al. Feasibility and Clinical Significance of In Vivo Cholesterol Crystal Detection Using Optical Coherence Tomography. Arterioscler Thromb Vasc Biol 2020;40:220–9.

39. Kataoka Y, Puri R, Hammadah M, et al. Cholesterol crystals associate with coronary plaque vulnerability in vivo. J Am Coll Cardiol 2015;65:630–2.

40. Shimokado A, Matsuo Y, Kubo T, et al. In vivo optical coherence tomography imaging and histopathology of healed coronary plaques. Atherosclerosis 2018;275:35–42.

41. Usui E, Mintz GS, Lee T, et al. Prognostic impact of healed coronary plaque in non-culprit lesions assessed by optical coherence tomography. Atherosclerosis 2020;309:1–7.

42. Fracassi F, Crea F, Sugiyama T, et al. Healed Culprit Plaques in Patients With Acute Coronary Syndromes. J Am Coll Cardiol 2019;73:2253–63.

43. Russo M, Kim HO, Kurihara O, et al. Characteristics of non-culprit plaques in acute coronary syndrome patients with layered culprit plaque. Eur Heart J Cardiovasc Imaging 2020;21:1421–30.

44. Okamoto H, Kume T, Yamada R, et al. Prevalence and Clinical Significance of Layered Plaque in Patients With Stable Angina Pectoris - Evaluation With Histopathology and Optical Coherence Tomography. Circ J 2019;83:2452–9.

45. Kurihara O, Russo M, Kim HO, et al. Clinical significance of healed plaque detected by optical coherence tomography: a 2-year follow-up study. J Thromb Thrombolysis 2020;50:895–902.

46. Usui E, Matsumura M, Mintz GS, et al. Clinical outcomes of low-intensity area without attenuation and cholesterol crystals in non-culprit lesions assessed by optical coherence tomography. Atherosclerosis 2021;332:41–7.

47. Uemura S, Ishigami K, Soeda T, et al. Thin-cap fibroatheroma and microchannel findings in optical coherence tomography correlate with subsequent progression of coronary atheromatous plaques. Eur Heart J 2012;33:78–85.

48. Araki M, Yonetsu T, Kurihara O, et al. Predictors of Rapid Plaque Progression: An Optical Coherence Tomography Study. JACC Cardiovasc Imaging 2021;14:1628–38.

49. Yamamoto MH, Yamashita K, Matsumura M, et al. Serial 3-Vessel Optical Coherence Tomography and Intravascular Ultrasound Analysis of Changing Morphologies Associated With Lesion Progression in Patients With Stable Angina Pectoris. Circ Cardiovasc Imaging 2017;10:e006347.

50. Xie Z, Hou J, Yu H, et al. Patterns of coronary plaque progression: phasic versus gradual. A combined optical coherence tomography and intravascular ultrasound study. Coron Artery Dis 2016;27:658–66.

51. Xing L, Higuma T, Wang Z, et al. Clinical Significance of Lipid-Rich Plaque Detected by Optical Coherence Tomography: A 4-Year Follow-Up Study. J Am Coll Cardiol 2017;69:2502–13.

52. Prati F, Romagnoli E, Gatto L, et al. Relationship between coronary plaque morphology of the left anterior descending artery and 12 months clinical outcome: the CLIMA study. Eur Heart J 2020;41:383–91.

53. Prati F, Gatto L, Fabbiocchi F, et al. Clinical outcomes of calcified nodules detected by optical coherence tomography: a sub-analysis of the CLIMA study. EuroIntervention 2020;16:380–6.

54. Akasaka T, Kubo T. OCT-derived coronary calcified nodules as a predictor of high-risk patients. EuroIntervention 2020;16:361–3.

55. Kubo T, Ino Y, Mintz GS, et al. Optical coherence tomography detection of vulnerable plaques at high risk of developing acute coronary syndrome. Eur Heart J Cardiovasc Imaging 2021;jeab028. https://doi.org/10.1093/ehjci/jeab028. Online ahead of print.

56. Kedhi E, Berta B, Roleder T, et al. Thin-cap fibroatheroma predicts clinical events in diabetic patients with normal fractional flow reserve: the COMBINE OCT-FFR trial. Eur Heart J 2021;42:4671–9.

57. Komukai K, Kubo T, Kitabata H, et al. Effect of atorvastatin therapy on fibrous cap thickness in coronary atherosclerotic plaque as assessed by optical coherence tomography: the EASY-FIT study. J Am Coll Cardiol 2014;64:2207–17.

58. Nicholls SJ, Kataoka Y, Nissen SE, et al. Effect of Evolocumab on Coronary Plaque Phenotype and Burden in Statin-Treated Patients Following Myocardial Infarction. JACC Cardiovasc Imaging 2022. https://doi.org/10.1016/j.jcmg.2022.03.002. S1936-878X(22)00143-00147.

59. Ono M, Kawashima H, Hara H, et al. Advances in IVUS/OCT and Future Clinical Perspective of Novel Hybrid Catheter System in Coronary Imaging. Front Cardiovasc Med 2020;7:119.

60. Muller J, Madder R. OCT-NIRS Imaging for Detection of Coronary Plaque Structure and Vulnerability. Front Cardiovasc Med 2020;7:90.

61. Ughi GJ, Wang H, Gerbaud E, et al. Clinical Characterization of Coronary Atherosclerosis With Dual-Modality OCT and Near-Infrared Autofluorescence Imaging. JACC Cardiovasc Imaging 2016;9:1304–14.

62. Chen X, Kim W, Serafino M, et al. Dual-modality optical coherence tomography and frequency-domain fluorescence lifetime imaging microscope system for intravascular imaging. J Biomed Opt 2020;25:096010.

Optical Coherence Tomography-Guided Percutaneous Coronary Intervention: Practical Application

Ziad A. Ali, MD, DPhil[a,b,*,1],
Keyvan Karimi Galougahi, MD, PhD[a,1],
Susan V. Thomas, MPH[a], Arsalan Abu-Much, MD[b],
Karen Chau, BS[a], Ali Dakroub, MD[a],
Evan S. Shlofmitz, DO[a], Allen Jeremias, MD, MSc[a,b],
Nick West, MD[c], Mitsuaki Matsumura, BS[b],
Gary S. Mintz, MD[b], Akiko Maehara, MD[b],
Richard A. Shlofmitz, MD[a]

KEYWORDS

- Optical coherence tomography (OCT) • Percutaneous coronary intervention (PCI)
- Intravascular ultrasound (IVUS) • Coronary atherosclerosis

KEY POINTS

- Optical coherence tomography (OCT) has greatly contributed to our understanding of the pathophysiollogy of coronary artery disease.
- A practical approach to OCT-guided percutaneous coronary intervention (PCI) may have hampered adoption.
- Systematic integration of OCT in daily practice, adhering to standardized diagnostic and treatment algorithms are essential to increase adoption and optimize PCI.

INTRODUCTION

Intravascular imaging by intravascular ultrasound (IVUS) and optical coherence tomography (OCT) enables detailed imaging of coronary arteries and provides valuable information that is complementary to angiography, which makes intravascular imaging an important adjunctive tool in percutaneous coronary intervention (PCI). Accumulating evidence from registries,[1–3] randomized controlled trials,[4,5] and meta-analyses[6,7]

showed an improvement in PCI outcomes with intravascular imaging guidance versus angiography guidance alone.

OCT uses near-infrared light emitted to and scattered from the vessel wall to generate high-resolution, cross-sectional, and three-dimensional images of vessels. As blood attenuates the OCT signal, flushing is required to remove blood during image acquisition. OCT has a greater axial resolution but lower penetration depth compared with IVUS, which limits OCT imaging, particularly in

[a] Department of Cardiology, St Francis Hospital, 100 Port Washington Boulevard, Roslyn, NY 11576, USA;
[b] Cardiovascular Research Foundation, 1700 Broadway, New York, NY 10029, USA; [c] Abbott Vascular, 3200 Lakeside Drive #5314, Santa Clara, CA 95054, USA
[1] Both authors contributed equally.
* Corresponding author. St Francis Hospital & Heart Center, 100 Port Washington Boulevard, Roslyn, NY 10528.
E-mail address: ziad.ali@dcvi.org
Twitter: @ziadalinyc (Z.A.A.)

the presence of highly attenuating structures such as red thrombus or lipid/necrotic core. Herein, we provide a concise practical guide for the use of intracoronary OCT during PCI.

OPTICAL COHERENCE TOMOGRAPHY IN PERCUTANEOUS CORONARY INTERVENTION

Practical Steps in Optical Coherence Tomography Image Acquisition

OCT imaging systems consist of an imaging catheter, a drive motor-operating control (DOC), and software. To set up OCT, the imaging catheter is attached to the purge syringe and flushed with the same material planned for coronary flushing, mostly radiocontrast and occasionally saline, to maintain consistency in the index of refraction. The catheter is then attached to the DOC. Intracoronary nitroglycerin is given before OCT imaging to dilate the vessel and prevent catheter-induced spasm. It is important to ensure that the guiding catheter is engaged at the coronary ostium for adequate clearance of the coronary artery and optimal image acquisition. Deep-seating of the guide is unnecessary and may be counter-productive as contrast injection may eject the guide, leading to sub-optimal flushing.

The OCT imaging steps can be remembered with the mnemonic four Ps: position, purge, puff, and pullback. The OCT catheter is advanced on the coronary guidewire and positioned distal to the target lesion, approximately ~10 mm distal to the target lesion, the catheter is again purged, and a small volume of flush is "puffed" through the guide catheter to evaluate clearance (if clearance is not adequate, guide catheter engagement should be corrected), and then pullback is activated. The contrast flush rate is set at 4 ml/s for a total volume of 14 to 16 ml for the left coronary artery and 3 ml/s for a total volume of 12 to 14 ml for the right coronary artery. If an automated injector is used, the pressure limit should be set at 300 psi. Contrast injection should be stopped as the guide catheter is seen on the pullback images to minimize contrast use. Cine angiography is performed during pullback to use contrast injection for angiography and for OCT coregistration if the feature is available. In severely stenotic lesions, if the OCT catheter does not cross the lesion or the vessel clearance is poor, predilatation should be performed to allow for image acquisition.

Percutaneous Coronary Intervention Guidance Using Optical Coherence Tomography

OCT images acquired before PCI can be used to assess lesion morphology to guide lesion

preparation strategies[8] and to identify stent landing zones with minimal or no disease. Precise measurements of vessel diameter and lesion length on the images can be used to select an appropriate balloon and stent sizes. Pre-PCI assessment with OCT can be summarized with the mnemonic MLD (Morphology, Length, and Diameter), whereas post-PCI assessment remembered as MAX (Medial dissection, Apposition, eXpansion), with the whole steps recalled as MLD MAX (Figs. 1–6). These parameters are inclusive of the procedural goals of PCI.

Pre-Percutaneous Coronary Intervention Guidance

Morphology: The trilaminar appearance represents the light scattering reflected from the layers of the normal vessel. In diseased vessels, there is a loss of this architecture, with morphologies that correlate with different types of atherosclerotic plaques. A simplified algorithm for OCT image interpretation is shown in Fig. 1. This algorithm is useful in describing the most frequent pathological morphologies. These morphologies in the vessel wall include low-attenuating, signal-rich lesions (fibrous plaques), high-attenuating, signal-poor regions covered with a fibrous cap (lipid-rich plaques), and low-attenuating, sharply delineated, signal-poor regions (calcific plaques). In the vessel lumen, low-attenuating white thrombus or high-attenuating red thrombus that casts a shadow on the vessel wall are the most common pathologies.

Assessment of lesion morphology on OCT can guide lesion preparation. Predilatation with an undersized balloon or direct stenting may be appropriate in fibrous or lipid-rich plaques, whereas in moderate or severely calcified lesions, noncompliant balloon predilatation, use of a cutting or scoring balloon, atherectomy or intravascular lithotripsy may be needed.

In calcified lesions, IVUS delineates the calcification arc but not the thickness because ultrasound waves reflect off calcium. In contrast, OCT allows for assessment of both calcification arc and thickness in most cases. An OCT-based scoring system has been devised and validated in calcified lesions to help determine which calcific morphologies lead to stent underexpansion.[9,10] These factors can be recalled as the "rule of 5s." Two points are given for maximum arc >50% of the circumference, 1 point for maximum thickness >0.5 mm, and 1 point for length >5 mm. There was significantly lower stent expansion in target lesions with a total score of 4 (all factors present), suggesting calcium modification with atherectomy or intravascular lithotripsy

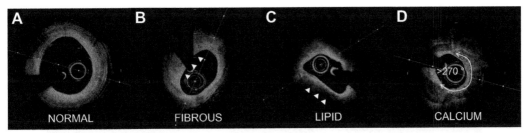

Fig. 1. Morphology. (*A*) The trilaminar appearance of the normal vessel or fibrous plaque represents light scattering reflecting from the layers of the vessel without light attenuation. (*B*) When the intima, media, and adventitia can be visualized for the whole vessel circumference, the cross-section may also represent a fibrous plaque differentiated by eccentric intimal thickening (*arrowheads*). The morphological characteristics of different plaque constituents hold different light-attenuating properties. High attenuation occurs when there is complete absorbance of the near infrared light, and low attenuation when the light is refracted, yet continues to allow visualization of vessel characteristics toward the adventitia. When the source of the attenuation is in the vessel wall, high attenuation represents (*C*) lipid (*arrowheads*), and low attenuation (*D*) calcium (*arrow*).

may be needed, whereas stent expansion in lesions with scores of 3 or less was generally acceptable. Calcium fracture using balloon angioplasty alone was best predicted by a calcium angle of 225° and calcium thickness of 0.24 mm.[11] In calcified lesions with a maximum calcium arc >50% of the vessel circumference, lesions with calcium fracture have better stent expansion than those without. Hence, the presence of calcium fracture, easily identified on OCT, may be a key goal of lesion preparation before stenting.

Length: OCT software provides a two-dimensional lumenogram of the artery referred to as the Lumen Profile, which incorporates multiplanar reconstruction of the three-dimensional data. To determine the lesion length, the sections with the largest lumen proximal to the lesion and distal to the lesion on the Lumen Profile are selected to create regions of interest. By scrolling through the OCT cross-sections at these regions, the most "normal" appearing segments, that is, segments where there are minimal atherosclerotic lesions and hence greatest visibility of the arterial medial (external

elastic lamina [EEL]) and adventitial layers, are selected as proximal and distal reference frames. The length of the lesion is automatically calculated by the OCT software (see Fig. 2). The lesion length usually does not correspond to the length of a commercially available DES. Therefore, either the proximal or distal reference frame, whichever is less diseased, is adjusted to an available DES length. This approach ensures minimizing stent edge problems, including geographic miss and the presence of thin-cap fibroatheroma (TCFA) at reference segments, which may lead to significant dissections and increase the risk of early stent thrombosis and post-PCI target lesion failure.[12–17]

Diameter: A step-by-step guide for the measurement of vessel diameter and selection of stent diameter is provided in Fig. 3. An EEL-guided sizing strategy is preferable to a lumen-guided strategy as it leads to the selection of relatively larger device sizes (≈0.5 mm) and, consequently, a larger lumen area without an increase in post-procedural complications.[18–20] EEL measurements may be used if two measurements can be made in vessel circumferences that

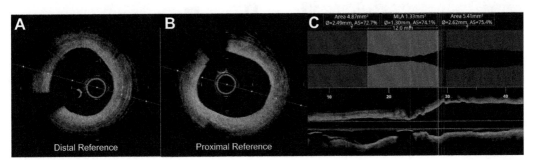

Fig. 2. Length. The reference segments should be perused to find normal (*A*) or fibrous (*B*) cross-sections. (*C*) The distance between the distal and proximal reference is automatically calculated in the OCT automated measures function (12 mm).

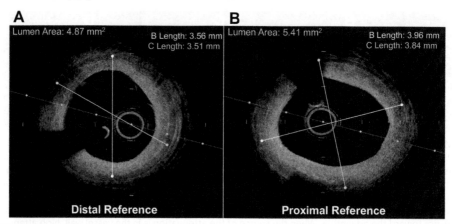

Fig. 3. Diameter. Vessel diameter should be assessed using the EEL-EEL diameter at the reference segments (rounding down to the nearest device size) unless the EEL cannot be identified, in which case luminal measures are used (rounded up between 0.25 and 0.5 mm to the nearest device size). In this case, the (A) distal reference measures 3.56 mm x 3.51 mm (mean 3.54 mm) using the EEL, and thus a 3.5 mm x 12 mm stent should be used. Based on the (B) proximal reference EEL-based measurements of 3.96 mm x 3.84 mm (mean 3.90 mm), a short 3.75 mm balloon may be used for post-dilation proximally. If the device is underexpanded distally after deployment, a 3.5 mm balloon should be used based on the distal reference sizing.

are at least one quadrant apart. Greater than 180° of EEL could be visualized in ~80% of cases in the ILUMIEN III trial.[19] EEL-based measurements should be rounded down, between 0.25 to 0.5 mm, to determine the device size. If EEL visibility is insufficient, the mean lumen diameter, recorded on the automated lumen profile feature, is used for device sizing. Lumen-based measurements should be rounded up between 0.25 and 0.5 mm, to determine the device size.[18] Distal measurements determine the stent size and distal post-dilation balloon and proximal measurements size of the proximal postdilation balloon.

Angiographic coregistration: A software for automated point-to-point correspondence between coronary angiogram and OCT frames has been developed that reduces the errors in the manual correlation of angiography with OCT cross-sections. The software allows for the selected distal and proximal landing sites on OCT to be marked on angiography to guide precise stent implantation. This feature allows for the prevention of landing the stent edges at angiographically normal appearing segments where plaque burden may be extensive.[21] In a randomized study, OCT-angiography coregistration aided in more precise stent deployment,

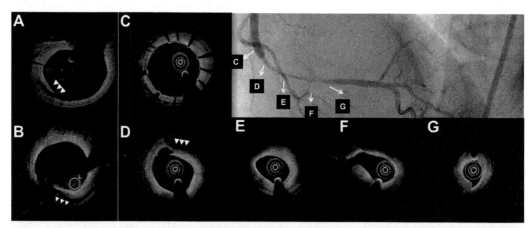

Fig. 4. Medial dissection. (A) Small intimal dissections that do not reach the media are most often benign and can be managed conservatively (arrowheads). (B) Dissections that reach the media (arrowheads) that are 3 mm long and greater than one quadrant in the arc are recommended for treatment with stent tacking, particularly if the dissection is distal. A representative case shows the (C) distal stent edge has a (D) medial dissection that progresses into an E–G intramural hematoma (arrowheads), causing luminal compromise.

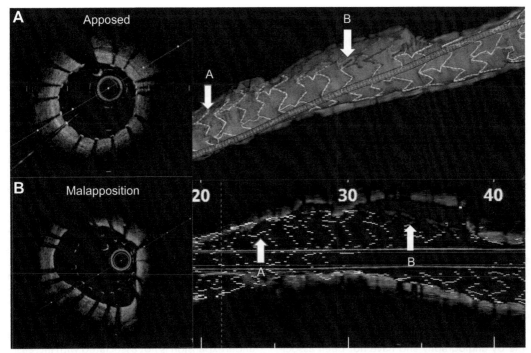

Fig. 5. Apposition. (A) A stent is apposed when the stent struts are in contact with the artery wall. (B) When the stent struts are not in contact with the vessel wall, this is malapposition. Treatment is recommended for malapposition when it is proximal, 3 mm in length, and gross, such that repeat attempts at wiring may cause inadvertent passage of the wire through stent struts.

eliminating large geographic miss (>5 mm), and resulted in a trend toward reducing major stent edge dissection compared with angiography guidance.[22] Similar findings were reported in observational studies reporting geographic miss with a length of ≈5 mm were identified on OCT in 70% of patients undergoing angiography-guided PCI,[23] with changes in the device landing zone and stent length with OCT guidance in ≈20% of patients compared with angiography-guided PCI.[24,25] OCT-angiography coregistration can also aid in quick identification and

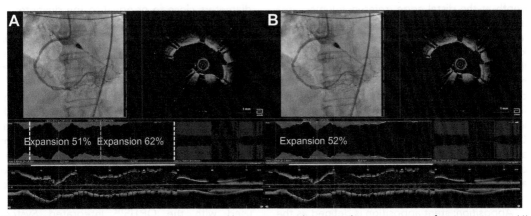

Fig. 6. Expansion. Stent expansion is determined by comparing the minimal stent area to a reference segment. (A) In the dual reference mode, the distal segment of the stent is compared with the distal reference cross-section located immediately outside the last stent frame, and the proximal segment of the stent is compared with the proximal reference cross-section located immediately before the first stent frame. (B) In the tapered reference mode, the expansion is calculated automatically based on interpolation of the expected vessel tapering that occurs with side branches, and underexpanded areas are automatically highlighted in red, whereas well-expanded areas are highlighted in white. Both techniques show significant stent underexpansion.

targeted postdilatation of under-expanded stent segments, thus avoiding unnecessary postdilatation, especially near stent edges where postdilatation may result in edge dissection.[26] The coregistration feature can also help in the identification of the side-branch ostium to minimize protrusion of stent struts into the main branch while ensuring full coverage of the ostium of the side-branch.[27]

Post-Percutaneous Coronary Intervention Guidance

After stent deployment, the steps to assess and optimize stent deployment and correct complications can be summarized with the mnemonic MAX:

Medial dissection: reference segments are assessed on post-PCI OCT pullback to check for medial dissection and intramural hematoma. The high resolution of OCT has been criticized for providing "too much" information, identifying dissections in up to 40% of PCIs.[19] Most (≈80%) of these dissections were not detectable by angiography and have not been associated with adverse clinical impact.[28] This is because most dissections detected by OCT heal without consequence following PCI.[17,29] Nevertheless, the presence of major stent edge dissection detected by OCT is a predictor of poor outcomes.[14–17] Data from registries suggest that major dissection, defined as a linear rim of tissue with a width >200 μm, at the distal but not proximal stent edge is associated with a 2.5-fold hazard of major adverse cardiovascular events (death, myocardial infarction, target lesion revascularization).[15,16] Moreover, cavity depth at the distal edge, reference lumen area at the proximal edge and overall dissection length are predictors of adverse events.[17] In keeping with these findings, the ongoing ILUMIEN IV randomized study categorizes major dissections as those with medial dissection ± intramural hematoma ≥60° in arc from the center of the vessel and/or ≥3 mm in length from the edge of the stent (see Fig. 4). Given the blinded OCT in the angiographic arm of this study, ILUMIEN IV should provide detailed insight into which edge dissections are associated with target vessel failure, thus needing correction.

Apposition: stent apposition is defined as the contact between stent struts and the vessel wall. Malapposition, that is, the lack of full apposition, may be present immediately after placement of stents (acute stent malapposition), or it may develop later (late stent malapposition). Late stent malapposition can be categorized as late persistent malapposition (ongoing since the time of stent implantation) or late acquired malapposition. Acute stent malapposition is a common finding after implantation of DES and is detected on average in half of the implanted stents OCT,[16] which is aided by the high resolution of OCT and the software that allows for automatic detection of malapposed struts. The potential impact, however, of acute stent malapposition on stent failure rates (ie, rates of in-stent restenosis and stent thrombosis) has been a matter of controversy.[30] Although in vitro data,[31] pathophysiological examination,[32] and small intravascular imaging studies[33] support a theoretical link between the exposed, uncovered malapposed struts and stent thrombosis; several larger intravascular imaging studies[15,34–36] have shown no relationship between the presence and extent of acute stent malapposition and early, late, or very late stent thrombosis or adverse events after DES implantation.[14–16,34–40]

Thus, acute stent malapposition without underexpansion is not associated with increased stent failure rates and does not need correction. Nevertheless, proximal malapposition that may interfere with re-wiring, gross malapposition for long segments (>3 mm), or malapposition associated with underexpansion would need correction (see Fig. 5). As the force required to appose struts is different from that required to expand them, noncompliant balloon inflation may not be necessary, and low-pressure inflation of semi-compliant balloons could be sufficient.

Expansion: if the stent expands the lesion to diameters close to or equal to the diameter of the artery, the stent is considered adequately expanded. The current European consensus is that a minimal stent area ≥80% of the mean reference lumen area and/or >4.5 mm^2 on OCT imaging is considered acceptable.[16,41] However, multiple criteria for adequate expansion have been proposed and tested,[41] with the common goal of maximizing the minimal stent area, a consistent predictor of long-term PCI outcomes.[3,42–48] OCT software provides automatic measurement of stent diameter and expansion and detection of underexpanded segments. For instance, the AptiVue™ software, used with the OPTIS™ Integrated System (Abbott), provides two modes of expansion assessment. The first mode is an automatic comparison of stent expansion to the closest respective proximal or distal reference segments in each half of the stent (Dual Reference mode), and the second is the automatic calculation of expansion based on interpolation of the vessel size, taking into account OCT-detected side branches (Tapered Reference mode) (see Fig. 6).

After stent underexpansion is identified on OCT and treated with high pressure (>18 atm) noncompliant balloon dilatation, vessel diameter at the segments immediately outside the stent edges are remeasured, using EEL-based measurements preferentially or lumen-guidance if the EEL is not visible. If the vessel size has not changed from the pre-PCI measurements to the post-PCI measurements, the operator has met their stent expansion optimization requirements pre-emptively, and further optimization for expansion is not warranted. If the vessel size has changed such that a new balloon diameter is recommended, postdilatation with noncompliant balloons sized to the target stent segment (EEL or lumen-based) should be performed to match the optimal expansion criteria. If the subsequent OCT run shows persistent underexpansion, further optimization would be at the discretion of the operator, considering the risk of complications such as perforation versus further gains in stent expansion.

Following OCT-guided optimization of stent expansion, the proximal and distal reference segments, defined as 5 mm from the edges of the stent, are examined for inflow/outflow disease. If both the proximal and distal reference segments have a minimal lumen area ≥4.5 mm^2, no further treatment is necessary. If there is untreated reference segment disease, defined as lumen area <4.5 mm^2 in either proximal or distal reference segments, an additional DES should be implanted unless anatomically prohibitive (eg, vessel tapering, distal diffuse disease, absence of a landing zone).

SUMMARY

Intravascular OCT provides high-resolution imaging data on coronary structures and pathologies, which can be systematically integrated into daily practice to optimize PCI. The current step-by-step guide provides operators with a practical manual on how to use OCT in coronary intervention. Although the current data support improved outcomes with IVUS-guided PCI compared with angiography-guided PCI, without difference in stent-related measures between OCT and IVUS guidance, the direct evidence for the potential clinical impact of OCT-guided PCI will be provided from the ongoing randomized trials, such as ILUMIEN IV study.

CLINICS CARE POINTS

- Injecting intracoronary nitroglycerin is highly advised to dilate the vessel and prevent catheter-induced spasm before optical coherence tomography (OCT) imaging.
- Deep intubation of the guide catheter is unnecessary as contrast injection may eject the guide, leading to suboptimal flushing.
- Remember the "4 Ps" of OCT imaging steps, position, purge, puff, and pullback.
- Target lesion "MLD" (Morphology, Length, and Diameter) is crucial for percutaneous coronary intervention planning.
- Mind the "MAX" (Medial dissection, Apposition, eXpansion) following stent deployment.

DISCLOSURE

The other authors have no conflicts of interest to declare.

ACKNOWLEDGMENTS

Z.A. Ali reports institutional research grants to St Francis Hospital from Abbott, Philips, Boston Scientific, Abiomed, Acist Medical, Medtronic, Cardiovascular Systems Inc., United States being a consultant to Amgen, AstraZeneca, and Boston Scientific, and having equity in Shockwave Medical. E.S. Shlofmitz: consultant for Abbott, Medtronic, Janssen Pharmaceuticals, OpSens Medical, Philips, and Shockwave. A. Jeremias: institutional funding (unrestricted education grant) from Philips/Volcano and is a consultant for Philips/Volcano, Abbott Vascular, United States, Acist Medical, and Boston Scientific. N. West: Employee of Abbott Vascular. G.S. Mintz reports honoraria from Abiomed, Boston Scientific, United States, Medtronic, and Philips, Netherlands. M. Matsumura is a consultant for Terumo and Boston Scientific. A. Maehara reports grant support from and being a consultant for Abbott Vascular and Boston Scientific. R.A. Shlofmitz reports speaker fees from Shockwave Medical.

REFERENCES

1. Maehara A, Mintz GS, Witzenbichler B, et al. Relationship between intravascular ultrasound guidance and clinical outcomes after drug-eluting stents. Circ Cardiovasc Interv 2018;11(11): e006243.
2. Jones DA, Rathod KS, Koganti S, et al. Angiography alone versus angiography plus optical coherence tomography to guide percutaneous

coronary intervention: outcomes from the Pan-London PCI cohort. JACC Cardiovasc Interv 2018; 11(14):1313–21.

3. Park H, Ahn JM, Kang DY, et al. Optimal stenting technique for complex coronary lesions: intracoronary imaging-guided pre-dilation, stent sizing, and post-dilation. JACC Cardiovasc Interv 2020; 13(12):1403–13.

4. Hong SJ, Mintz GS, Ahn CM, et al. Effect of intravascular ultrasound-guided drug-eluting stent implantation: 5-year follow-up of the IVUS-XPL randomized trial. JACC Cardiovasc Interv 2020;13(1):62–71.

5. Zhang J, Gao X, Kan J, et al. Intravascular ultrasound versus angiography-guided drug-eluting stent implantation: the ULTIMATE trial. J Am Coll Cardiol 2018;72(24):3126–37.

6. di Mario C, Koskinas KC, Räber L. Clinical benefit of IVUS guidance for coronary stenting: the ULTIMATE step toward definitive evidence? J Am Coll Cardiol 2018;72(24):3138–41.

7. Elgendy IY, Mahmoud AN, Elgendy AY, et al. Intravascular ultrasound-guidance is associated with lower cardiovascular mortality and myocardial infarction for drug-eluting stent implantation - insights from an updated meta-analysis of randomized trials. Circ J 2019;83(6):1410–3.

8. Raber L, Mintz GS, Koskinas KC, et al. Clinical use of intracoronary imaging. Part 1: guidance and optimization of coronary interventions. an expert consensus document of the European Association of Percutaneous Cardiovascular Interventions. Eur Heart J 2018;14(6):656–77.

9. Fujino A, Mintz GS, Matsumura M, et al. A new optical coherence tomography-based calcium scoring system to predict stent underexpansion. EuroIntervention 2018;13(18):e2182–9.

10. Ali ZA, Galougahi KK. Shining light on calcified lesions, plaque stabilisation and physiologic significance: new insights from intracoronary OCT. EuroIntervention 2018;13(18):e2105–8.

11. Fujino A, Mintz GS, Lee T, et al. Predictors of calcium fracture derived from balloon angioplasty and its effect on stent expansion assessed by optical coherence tomography. JACC Cardiovasc Interv 2018;11(10):1015–7.

12. Ino Y, Kubo T, Matsuo Y, et al. Optical coherence tomography predictors for edge restenosis after everolimus-eluting stent implantation. Circ Cardiovasc Interv 2016;9(10):e004231.

13. Prati F, Kodama T, Romagnoli E, et al. Suboptimal stent deployment is associated with subacute stent thrombosis: optical coherence tomography insights from a multicenter matched study. From the CLI Foundation investigators: the CLI-THRO study. Am Heart J 2015;169(2):249–56.

14. Prati F, Romagnoli E, Gatto L, et al. Clinical impact of suboptimal stenting and residual intrastent

plaque/thrombus protrusion in patients with acute coronary syndrome: the CLI-OPCI ACS substudy (centro per la lotta contro l'infarto-optimization of percutaneous coronary intervention in acute coronary syndrome). Circ Cardiovasc Interv 2016;9(12): e003726.

15. Prati F, Romagnoli E, La Manna A, et al. Long-term consequences of optical coherence tomography findings during percutaneous coronary intervention: the Centro Per La Lotta Contro L'infarto - Optimization Of Percutaneous Coronary Intervention (CLI-OPCI) LATE study. EuroIntervention 2018; 14(4):e443–51.

16. Prati F, Romagnoli E, Burzotta F, et al. Clinical impact of OCT findings during PCI: the CLI-OPCI II Study. JACC Cardiovasc Imaging 2015;8(11): 1297–305.

17. van Zandvoort LJC, Tomaniak M, Tovar Forero MN, et al. Predictors for clinical outcome of untreated stent edge dissections as detected by optical coherence tomography. Circ Cardiovasc Interv 2020;13(3):e008685.

18. Shlofmitz E, Jeremias A, Parviz Y, et al. External elastic lamina vs. luminal diameter measurement for determining stent diameter by optical coherence tomography: an ILUMIEN III substudy. Eur Heart J Cardiovasc Imaging 2020;22(7):753–9.

19. Ali ZA, Maehara A, Genereux P, et al. Optical coherence tomography compared with intravascular ultrasound and with angiography to guide coronary stent implantation (ILUMIEN III: OPTIMIZE PCI): a randomised controlled trial. Lancet 2016; 388(10060):2618–28.

20. Kubo T, Shinke T, Okamura T, et al. Optical frequency domain imaging vs. intravascular ultrasound in percutaneous coronary intervention (OPINION trial): one-year angiographic and clinical results. Eur Heart J 2017;38(42):3139–47.

21. Mintz GS, Painter JA, Pichard AD, et al. Atherosclerosis in angiographically "normal" coronary artery reference segments: an intravascular ultrasound study with clinical correlations. J Am Coll Cardiol 1995;25(7):1479–85.

22. Koyama K, Fujino A, Maehara A, et al. A prospective, single-center, randomized study to assess whether automated coregistration of optical coherence tomography with angiography can reduce geographic miss. Catheter Cardiovasc Interv 2019;93(3):411–8.

23. Hebsgaard L, Nielsen TM, Tu S, et al. Co-registration of optical coherence tomography and X-ray angiography in percutaneous coronary intervention. the Does Optical Coherence Tomography Optimize Revascularization (DOCTOR) fusion study. Int J Cardiol 2015;182:272–8.

24. Leistner DM, Riedel M, Steinbeck L, et al. Real-time optical coherence tomography coregistration with

angiography in percutaneous coronary intervention-impact on physician decision-making: the OPTICO-integration study. Catheter Cardiovasc Interv 2018; 92(1):30–7.

25. Schneider VS, Böhm F, Blum K, et al. Impact of real-time angiographic co-registered optical coherence tomography on percutaneous coronary intervention: the OPTICO-integration II trial. Clin Res Cardiol 2021;110(2):249–57.

26. Romagnoli E, Sangiorgi GM, Cosgrave J, et al. Drug-eluting stenting: the case for post-dilation. JACC Cardiovasc Interv 2008;1(1):22–31.

27. Shlofmitz E, Sosa F, Goldberg A, et al. Bifurcation and ostial optical coherence tomography mapping (BOOM) - case description of a novel bifurcation stent technique. Cardiovasc Revasc Med 2018; 19(8s):47–9.

28. Chamié D, Bezerra HG, Attizzani GF, et al. Incidence, predictors, morphological characteristics, and clinical outcomes of stent edge dissections detected by optical coherence tomography. JACC Cardiovasc Interv 2013;6(8):800–13.

29. Radu MD, Räber L, Heo J, et al. Natural history of optical coherence tomography-detected non-flow-limiting edge dissections following drug-eluting stent implantation. EuroIntervention 2014; 9(9):1085–94.

30. Mintz GS. Why are we so concerned with acute incomplete stent apposition? Eur Heart J Cardiovasc Imaging 2015;16(1):110–1.

31. Foin N, Lu S, Ng J, et al. Stent malapposition and the risk of stent thrombosis: mechanistic insights from an in vitro model. EuroIntervention 2017; 13(9):e1096–8.

32. Joner M, Finn AV, Farb A, et al. Pathology of drug-eluting stents in humans: delayed healing and late thrombotic risk. J Am Coll Cardiol 2006;48(1): 193–202.

33. Ozaki Y, Okumura M, Ismail TF, et al. The fate of incomplete stent apposition with drug-eluting stents: an optical coherence tomography-based natural history study. Eur Heart J 2010;31(12):1470–6.

34. Wang B, Mintz GS, Witzenbichler B, et al. Predictors and long-term clinical impact of acute stent malapposition: an assessment of dual antiplatelet therapy with drug-eluting stents (ADAPT-DES) intravascular ultrasound substudy. J Am Heart Assoc 2016;5(12):e004438.

35. Steinberg DH, Mintz GS, Mandinov L, et al. Long-term impact of routinely detected early and late incomplete stent apposition: an integrated intravascular ultrasound analysis of the TAXUS IV, V, and VI and TAXUS ATLAS workhorse, long lesion, and direct stent studies. JACC Cardiovasc Interv 2010;3(5):486–94.

36. Im E, Kim BK, Ko YG, et al. Incidences, predictors, and clinical outcomes of acute and late stent malapposition detected by optical coherence tomography after drug-eluting stent implantation. Circ Cardiovasc Interv 2014;7(1):88–96.

37. Guo N, Maehara A, Mintz GS, et al. Incidence, mechanisms, predictors, and clinical impact of acute and late stent malapposition after primary intervention in patients with acute myocardial infarction: an intravascular ultrasound substudy of the Harmonizing Outcomes with Revascularization and Stents in Acute Myocardial Infarction (HORIZONS-AMI) trial. Circulation 2010;122(11): 1077–84.

38. Romagnoli E, Gatto L, La Manna A, et al. Role of residual acute stent malapposition in percutaneous coronary interventions. Catheter Cardiovasc Interv 2017;90(4):566–75.

39. van der Hoeven BL, Liem SS, Dijkstra J, et al. Stent malapposition after sirolimus-eluting and bare-metal stent implantation in patients with ST-segment elevation myocardial infarction: acute and 9-month intravascular ultrasound results of the MISSION! intervention study. JACC Cardiovasc Interv 2008;1(2):192–201.

40. Soeda T, Uemura S, Park SJ, et al. Incidence and clinical significance of poststent optical coherence tomography findings: one-year follow-up study from a multicenter registry. Circulation 2015; 132(11):1020–9.

41. Räber L, Mintz GS, Koskinas KC, et al. Clinical use of intracoronary imaging. part 1: guidance and optimization of coronary interventions. an expert consensus document of the European Association of Percutaneous Cardiovascular Interventions. Eur Heart J 2018;39(35):3281–300.

42. Choi SY, Maehara A, Cristea E, et al. Usefulness of minimum stent cross sectional area as a predictor of angiographic restenosis after primary percutaneous coronary intervention in acute myocardial infarction (from the HORIZONS-AMI Trial IVUS substudy). Am J Cardiol 2012;109(4): 455–60.

43. Hong SJ, Kim BK, Shin DH, et al. Effect of intravascular ultrasound-guided vs angiography-guided everolimus-eluting stent implantation: the IVUS-XPL randomized clinical trial. JAMA 2015;314(20): 2155–63.

44. Kang J, Cho YS, Kim SW, et al. Intravascular ultrasound and angiographic predictors of in-stent restenosis of chronic total occlusion lesions. PLoS One 2015;10(10):e0140421.

45. Kang SJ, Ahn JM, Song H, et al. Comprehensive intravascular ultrasound assessment of stent area and its impact on restenosis and adverse cardiac events in 403 patients with unprotected left main disease. Circ Cardiovasc Interv 2011;4(6):562–9.

46. Song HG, Kang SJ, Ahn JM, et al. Intravascular ultrasound assessment of optimal stent area to

prevent in-stent restenosis after zotarolimus-, ever-olimus-, and sirolimus-eluting stent implantation. Catheter Cardiovasc Interv 2014;83(6):873–8.

47. Lee SY, Shin DH, Kim JS, et al. Intravascular ultra-sound predictors of major adverse cardiovascular events after implantation of everolimus-eluting

stents for long coronary lesions. Rev Esp Cardiol (Engl Ed) 2017;70(2):88–95.

48. Katagiri Y, De Maria GL, Kogame N, et al. Impact of post-procedural minimal stent area on 2-year clin-ical outcomes in the SYNTAX II trial. Catheter Cardiovasc Interv 2019;93(4):E225–34.

Optical Coherence Tomography-Guided Percutaneous Coronary Intervention: Evidence and Clinical Trials

Hiromasa Otake, MD, PhD

KEYWORDS

• Optical coherence tomography • Intravascular ultrasound • Coronary intervention • PCI

KEY POINTS

- Optical coherence tomography (OCT) is superior to intravascular ultrasound (IVUS) in terms of the precision of quantitative and qualitative intracoronary evaluation.
- OCT is useful to guide percutaneous coronary intervention (PCI) in cases of lipid-rich plaque and severely calcified plaque.
- Clinical trials have shown that OCT-guided PCI is superior to angiography-guided PCI with respect to acute procedural results and noninferior to IVUS-guided PCI with respect to acute procedural results and mid-term clinical outcomes.
- The benefits of intracoronary imaging depend largely on the interpretation and the operators' reaction to the findings; hence, operators should acquaint themselves with several important pieces of evidence regarding OCT-guided PCI.

INTRODUCTION

Percutaneous coronary intervention (PCI) is an established treatment for patients with coronary artery disease. Since its discovery, coronary angiography has been essential for guiding PCI procedures; however, angiography can only visualize intracoronary lumina in a two-dimensional manner. Unlike angiography, intravascular ultrasound (IVUS) can provide direct information on atherosclerosis and other pathologic conditions within the vessel wall that can misguide operators during catheter-based interventions. Unlike angiography, IVUS directly visualizes atherosclerosis and other pathologic conditions within the vessel wall. With its user-friendliness and ability to visualize the entire arterial cross-section in real time, IVUS has become the most widely used intravascular imaging modality

during PCI. In recent clinical trials, it has been shown that IVUS offers significant improvements in clinical outcomes after PCI using second-generation drug-eluting stents.

Optical coherence tomography (OCT) is an intravascular imaging modality that allows for detailed microstructural evaluation during PCI. With this unique feature, it has become widely used as an adjunctive imaging tool for PCI. Recently, several studies have shown a significant advantage of OCT-guided PCI in several specific situations. Furthermore, several clinical trials have evaluated the superiority and noninferiority of OCT-guided PCI as compared with angiography-guided PCI and IVUS-guided PCI, respectively. This article summarizes the data supporting the application of OCT-guided PCI to several specific situations, introduces essential evidence, and discusses the ongoing

---

Division of Cardiovascular Medicine, Department of Internal Medicine, Kobe University Graduate School of Medicine, 7-5-1 Kusunoki-cho, Chuo-ku, Kobe, Hyogo 650-0017, Japan
E-mail address: hotake@med.kobe-u.ac.jp

Intervent Cardiol Clin 12 (2023) 225–236
https://doi.org/10.1016/j.iccl.2022.12.004
2211-7458/23/© 2023 Elsevier Inc. All rights reserved.

controversies and limitations in the context of the current evidence in the field of OCT-guided PCI.

EVIDENCE
Quantitative Analysis by Optical Coherence Tomography
Regarding OCT-guided PCI, the accuracy of measurements for quantitative analysis is vital. Since the resolution of OCT is more than 10 times higher than that of IVUS, it has been recognized as one of the most precise intravascular imaging modalities available. In the previous OPUS-CLASS trial, the mean lumen area according to Fourier domain (FD)-OCT was equal to the actual lumen area of the phantom model with low standard deviation. IVUS overestimated the lumen area and was less reproducible than FD-OCT (8.03 ± 0.58 mm^2 vs 7.45 ± 0.17 mm^2; $P < 0.001$).[1] In a recent head-to-head comparison of quantitative measurements between contemporary intravascular imaging systems, the accuracy of quantitative measurements among optical frequency domain imaging (OFDI), FD-OCT, and 6 mechanically rotating IVUS systems were evaluated in an in vitro phantom model.[2] All the imaging systems showed good accuracy and excellent precision of luminal measurements, with the relative differences between the measured diameter and actual phantom diameter ranging from −2.9% to 8.0% and minimum standard deviations of the measured diameters (≤ 0.02 mm). In addition, Garcia-Guimaraes and colleagues[3] showed that 60-MHz, high-definition IVUS (HD-IVUS) had excellent concordance with FD-OCT on quantitative measurements both before and after stent implantation. These findings imply that comparable stent expansion could be obtained via contemporary IVUS and OCT imaging if similar stent sizing protocols are applied.

Qualitative Analysis by Optical Coherence Tomography
In a pathological study, Yabushita and colleagues[4] introduced objective OCT image criteria for differentiating distinct components of atherosclerotic tissue in vitro and showed high accuracy for diagnosing plaque types based on the correlation of OCT images of 357 (diseased) atherosclerotic arterial segments from autopsies with histological analysis; in the histological analysis, OCT images of fibrous plaques were characterized by homogeneous, signal-rich regions; fibrocalcific plaques by well-delineated, signal-poor regions with sharp borders; and lipid-rich plaques by signal-poor

regions with diffuse borders. Independent validation of these criteria by 2 OCT readers showed a sensitivity and specificity ranging from 71% to 79% and 97% to 98% for fibrous plaques, 95% to 96% and 97% for fibrocalcific plaques, and 90% to 94% and 90% to 92% for lipid-rich plaques, respectively (overall agreement, $\kappa = 0.83$ to 0.84). The interobserver and intraobserver reliabilities of OCT assessment were high (κ values of 0.88 and 0.91, respectively). This unique ability of OCT to accurately diagnose plaque characteristics, including the presence of lipid and calcification, has helped build the treatment strategy for PCI.

Lipid plaque
The presence of a lipid plaque is one of the features that should be monitored during PCI. Similar to the presence of plaque rupture, attenuated signal plaque, and lipid pool-like image by IVUS, the extent of lipid components in the culprit plaque and the presence of thin-cap fibroatheroma (TCFA) are considered potential risk factors for periprocedural complications of PCI. Tanaka and colleagues[5] showed that an increase in the lipid arc at non-ST-elevation myocardial infarction culprit lesions was an independent predictor for the occurrence of the no-reflow phenomenon. In this study, the prevalence of TCFA was significantly higher in the no-reflow group than in the reflow group (50% vs 16%, $P = 0.005$). Several other investigators confirmed these relations using different approaches. Lee and colleagues[6] showed that OCT-derived TCFA was associated with post-PCI cardiac troponin I elevation in patients with elective stent implantation. They reported that the presence of OCT-derived TCFA was an independent predictor of post-PCI myocardial infarction after stenting (odds ratio [OR] 10.47; 95% confidence interval [CI] 3.74–29.28; $P < 0.001$). Ozaki and colleagues[7] showed that OCT-derived TCFA was more frequently detected in patients with microvascular obstruction as estimated by magnetic resonance imaging after PCI for patients with the acute coronary syndrome (ACS) (43% vs 9%, $P = 0.012$). A representative case with no-reflow phenomenon is summarized in Fig. 1.

The impact of a lipid plaque is not limited to periprocedural complications but also PCI-related complications in the chronic phase. In a retrospective study enrolling a total of 319 patients who underwent OCT immediately after everolimus-eluting stent implantation, Ino and colleagues[8] showed that lipidic plaques (OR 5.99; 95% CI 2.89–12.81; $P < 0.001$) and

A Before stenting   **B** After stenting

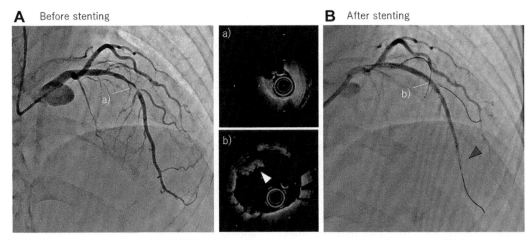

Fig. 1. A representative case of lipid-rich plaque and TCFA, leading to no-reflow phenomenon (*A*) Before stenting: (a) lipid-rich plaque with thin-cap fibroatheroma (TCFA). (*B*) After stenting: red arrowhead indicates no-reflow phenomenon, (b) post-stent OCT image with plaque protrusion (*white arrowhead*).

minimum lumen area (OR 0.64; 95% CI 0.42–0.96; $P = 0.029$) were independent predictors of binary stent-edge restenosis. Receiver operating characteristic analysis showed that a lipid arc of 185° (sensitivity 71%; specificity 72%; area under the curve [AUC] 0.761) and minimum lumen area of 4.10 mm^2 (sensitivity 67%; specificity 77%; AUC 0.787) were optimal cutoff values for predicting ischemia-driven binary stent-edge restenosis. This information is useful from a practical perspective, especially in diffuse long lesions wherein detecting optimal landing zones is often challenging.

Calcified lesions

PCI for severely calcified lesions remains challenging because of difficulties with balloon/stent delivery and achieving optimal stent expansion. This can be associated with an increased rate of procedural failure and suboptimal postprocedural outcomes compared to PCI for non-calcified lesions. OCT is one of the most effective tools to guide PCI for calcified lesions since it facilitates the evaluation of severity of calcification based on the longitudinal and circumferential calcium distributions and its accurate thickness measurements.

In a previous retrospective study of 61 patients with a heavily calcified culprit lesion on coronary angiography, Kubo and colleagues[9] studied the relationship between the thickness of calcium fracture, calcium fracture after balloon angioplasty, and extent of stent expansion. They reported that the median and maximal calcium fracture thickness were 450 μm (interquartile range, 300 to 660 μm) and 770 μm, respectively. They also reported

that lesions with calcium fracture were associated with better stent expansion and lower incidence of ischemia-driven target lesion revascularization (7% vs 28%; $P = 0.046$) than those without. These findings were confirmed by Maejima and colleagues,[10] who evaluated the relationship between OCT-based calcium findings after rotational atherectomy (RA) and calcium crack development after adjunctive balloon angioplasty. They reported that segments with calcium cracks after angioplasty had a larger median calcium arc (360°, IQR 246°–360° vs 147°, IQR 118°–199°; $P < 0.001$) and thinner calcium thickness (0.53 ± 0.28 mm vs 1.02 ± 0.42 mm; $P < 0.001$) than those without. The optimal thresholds of calcium arc and calcium thickness for prediction of cracks were 227° and 0.67 mm, respectively. These data indicate the need for optimal lesion preparation in treating heavily calcified lesions, and that OCT could be a powerful tool to speculate the probability of the formation of calcium crack with optimal dilatation without RA ablation.

RA is a potential treatment option for severely calcified lesions that can effectively ablate calcified plaques, thereby facilitating balloon/stent delivery and optimal stent expansion. However, complications associated with RA procedures have been reported, such as perforation, slow-flow/no-reflow phenomenon, and coronary artery dissection. In addition, insufficient atherectomy for calcification might lead to future in-stent restenosis due to insufficient stent expansion. Therefore, intravascular imaging might be recommended before RA to avoid potential procedure-related complications and to achieve effective RA ablation. In a recent retrospective study of 25 patients (26 lesions) who underwent OFDI before and after RA, we evaluated whether RA location and area in calcified plaque could be predicted using pre-RA OFDI and investigated associated predictive factors.[11] Consequently, we reported that in 87% of cross-sections, at least part of the predicted region—the region where a circle, similar in size to that of the Rota burr used, drawn in the center of the OFDI catheter overlapped the vessel wall—was ablated. Therefore, we considered that RA location can be somehow predicted using the OFDI catheter pathway. Conversely, when taking the area into consideration, the median %Correct- (how correct the predicted area was) and %Error-areas (the area that was unexpectedly ablated) were 43.1% and 64.2%, respectively. This suggested that the accuracy of OFDI catheter-based prediction for the amount of ablation was not high. In this study, floppy wire use, narrow lumen area, OFDI catheter close to the intima, and large arc of calcium were independently associated with a good prediction (high %Correct-/low %Error-areas). Conversely, in addition to non-left anterior descending lesions and OFDI catheter/wire far from the intima, the OFDI catheter far from the wire was associated with poor prediction of the ablated area (low %Correct-/high %Error-areas). This finding suggests that the errors may be, in part, attributable to the fundamental difference in catheter designs between the Rota burr and OFDI catheter (i.e., over-the-wire vs short-monorail rapid-exchange configurations). Since the Rota burr passes over the wire, wire-based, rather than OFDI catheter-based, predictions might be helpful if the OFDI catheter and guidewire are far apart (Fig. 2). Representative cases of good prediction and poor prediction are shown in Fig. 3.

Clinical Trials
Optical coherence tomography-guided percutaneous coronary intervention in the general population
Several clinical trials have evaluated the impact of OCT-guided PCI as compared with angiography- or IVUS-guided PCI. In 2012, Prati and colleagues[12] reported the results of a large-scale multicenter retrospective registry comparing angiographic plus OCT guidance versus angiographic guidance alone for routine PCI. Unadjusted analyses at mid-term follow-up showed that the OCT group had a significantly lower 12-month risk of cardiac death (1.2% vs 4.5%; P = 0.010), cardiac death or MI (6.6% vs 13.0%; P = 0.006), and a composite of cardiac

death, MI, or repeat revascularization (9.6% vs 14.8%; P = 0.044). Despite adjusting for baseline and procedural differences between the groups with multivariable logistic regression analysis and propensity score-adjusted analysis, OCT guidance remained associated with a significantly lower risk of cardiac death or MI. These findings were confirmed by a larger scale cohort study (Pan-London PCI registry), which included 123,764 patients who underwent PCI in National Health Service hospitals in London.[13] A significant difference in mortality was observed between patients who underwent OCT-guided PCI (7.7%) compared with patients who underwent either IVUS-guided (12.2%) or angiography-guided (15.7%; P < 0.0001) PCI, with differences seen for both elective (P < 0.0001) and ACS subgroups (P = 0.0024). Overall, this difference persisted after multivariate Cox analysis (hazard ratio [HR] 0.48; 95% CI 0.26 to 0.81; P = 0.001) and propensity matching (HR 0.39; 95% CI 0.21 to 0.77; P = 0.0008 for OCT vs angiography-alone cohorts), with no difference in matched OCT and IVUS cohorts (HR 0.88; 95% CI 0.61 to 1.38; P = 0.43). These data from large-scale registries implied better clinical outcomes in OCT-guided PCI than in angiography-guided PCI with clinical outcomes similar to those with IVUS-guided PCI.

Habara and colleagues[14] reported the results of the first randomized study in this field by enrolling 70 patients with de novo coronary lesions to compare OCT-guided versus IVUS-guided PCI. The primary endpoint of minimum stent area (MSA) was significantly larger with IVUS guidance than with OCT guidance (7.1 ± 2.1 mm^2 vs 6.1 ± 2.2 mm^2, respectively). In this study, they also reported that, compared with OCT imaging, IVUS imaging had a significantly better vessel border visibility at the most stenotic and reference segments. They speculated that difficulties in vessel border detection via OCT were reflected in lower deployment pressure as well as lower frequency and pressure of post-balloon dilatation in the OCT-guided PCI group, resulting in a significantly smaller MSA achieved post-PCI. However, owing to small numbers of patients, these results were hypothesis generating, and this study was not sufficiently powered to evaluate the clinical outcomes of OCT-guided PCI as compared with IVUS-guided PCI.

In 2016, two large-scale, prospective, randomized studies were conducted to evaluate the efficacy of OCT-guided PCI as compared with IVUS- or angiography-guided PCI. The ILUMIEN III study was a prospective, randomized,

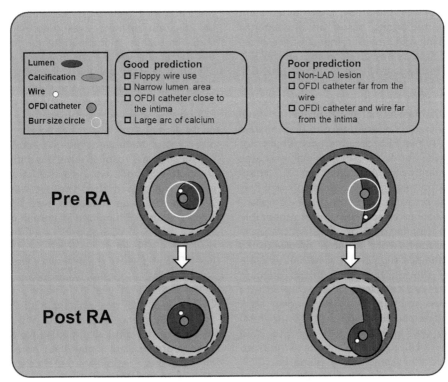

Fig. 2. Associated factors to predict rotational atherectomy location. Floppy wire use, narrow lumen area, OFDI catheter close to the intima, and large arc of calcium are independently associated with good prediction. Non-left anterior descending (LAD) lesions, OFDI catheter far from the wire, and OFDI catheter and wire far from the intima are associated with poor prediction by OFDI.

multicenter trial designed to compare the efficacy and safety of OCT guidance to IVUS guidance and angiographic guidance.[15] The primary efficacy and safety endpoints were final post-PCI MSA measured by OCT and procedural MACE, respectively. A total of 450 patients were randomized to OCT guidance, IVUS guidance, or angiography-guided stent implantation

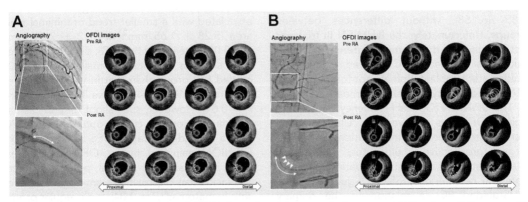

Fig. 3. Representative angiography and OFDI of good and poor prediction cases. (A) Good prediction case. (B) Poor prediction case. Angiography images with (upper left) and without contrast (lower left) are shown. OFDI results before and after RA are shown (right). White double-head arrow indicates target lesions. White triangles indicate wire position. White circles indicate the circle with Rota burr dimensions. Blue dotted line indicates the predicted ablation area (P-area). Yellow dotted line indicates the actual ablation area (A-area). The green dotted area indicates the P-area with wire-based prediction. In the good prediction case (A), P-area and A-area are similar in all cross-sections, whereas in the poor prediction case, A-area is located around the wire position on the pre-RA OFDI image (green dotted area) and not around the OFDI catheter (blue dotted line: P-area). A-area, real ablation area; OFDI, optical frequency domain imaging; P-area, predicted ablation area; RA, rotational atherectomy.

in a 1:1:1 ratio. In this study, OCT-guided stent sizing was performed based on the external elastic lamina (EEL) measurements of the proximal and distal reference segments. If the EEL circumference was available for >180°, the EEL diameter was accepted as the vessel size. Next, the stent diameter was chosen by the smaller EEL diameter of the proximal or distal reference and rounded down to the nearest 0.25-mm. If the EEL circumference could not be visualized for >180°, lumen diameter was used for stent sizing. After stenting, OCT imaging was performed, if necessary, along with iterative high-pressure or larger non-compliant balloon inflations to achieve at least acceptable stent expansion (an MSA of >90% in both proximal and distal halves of the stent relative to the closest reference segment). Based on this criterion, they showed that OCT-guided stenting achieved an MSA similar to that achieved with IVUS-guided stenting. The final median MSA was 5.79 (first and third quartiles, 4.54 to 7.34) mm^2 after OCT guidance, 5.89 (4.67 to 7.80) mm^2 after IVUS guidance, and 5.49 (4.39 to 6.59) mm^2 after angiography guidance. OCT guidance showed an MSA similar to that achieved with angiography guidance ($P = 0.12$) but had a significantly greater stent expansion than that achieved with angiography guidance ($P = 0.02$). Furthermore, OCT guidance was noninferior ($P = 0.001$) but not superior to IVUS guidance with respect to MSA post-PCI ($P = 0.42$). OCT guidance also resulted in fewer cases of major dissection and major malapposition than those with IVUS guidance and angiography guidance. Overall procedural MACE was 3.8% (6/158), without differences between groups. Unfortunately, the ILUMIEN III trial was not designed to detect the difference in clinical outcomes between OCT-guided and IVUS-guided stent implantation except for procedural MACE and 30-day clinical outcomes.

The OPINION (Optical Frequency Domain Imaging [OFDI] vs Intravascular Ultrasound in Percutaneous Coronary Intervention) trial is the largest prospective, multicenter, randomized trial to date, and included 829 patients to evaluate the noninferiority of OFDI-guided PCI to IVUS-guided PCI in relation to the primary endpoint of target vessel failure (a composite of cardiac death, target vessel-related myocardial infarction, and ischemia-driven target vessel revascularization) at 1 year.[16] To date, this is the only randomized trial to evaluate the efficacy of OCT-guided PCI as compared with IVUS-guided PCI in terms of the clinical endpoint 1 year after PCI. Unlike the ILUMIEN III trial, the OPINION

trial adopted reference lumen-based stent sizing. Stent diameter was determined as 0–0.25 mm greater than mean lumen diameter at the distal reference site followed by post-dilatation using a balloon with diameter of 0–0.25 mm greater than mean lumen diameter at the proximal reference site; in the IVUS-guided PCI group, however, stent diameter was determined as equal or larger, and smaller than the mean vessel diameter at the distal and proximal reference sites, respectively. This difference in stent sizing criteria was reflected in the difference in the chosen stent size between groups. The selected stent diameter was significantly smaller in the OFDI-guided PCI group compared with the IVUS-guided PCI group (2.92 ± 0.39 mm vs 2.99 ± 0.39 mm; $P = 0.005$); however, the difference was minimal. Nevertheless, the primary endpoint of target vessel failure at 1 year in patients undergoing OFDI-guided PCI was noninferior to that in patients undergoing IVUS-guided PCI (5.2% vs 4.9%; P for noninferiority = 0.04). No difference in angiographic late lumen loss, percent diameter stenosis, or binary restenosis rate was observed at 8 months.

The OPINION trial had its own pre-specified imaging substudy to clarify how IVUS- and OCT-guidance affect PCI in terms of acute and mid-term vessel reaction after current-generation drug-eluting stent implantation.[17] A total of 103 initial consecutive patients were enrolled into this substudy, and all patients were imaged using both modalities (IVUS and OFDI) after PCI, and via OFDI at 8 months. Immediately after PCI, OFDI-guided PCI was associated with a smaller trend of minimal stent area (5.28 ± 1.65 mm^2 vs 6.12 ± 2.34 mm^2; $P = 0.088$) measured by OFDI, since the selected stent size was significantly smaller in the OFDI-guided PCI group than that in the IVUS-guided PCI group (2.92 ± 0.41 mm vs 3.11 ± 0.39 mm; $P = 0.01$). However, such slight differences had no influence on the clinical outcomes after PCI with a second-generation DES as shown in the OPINION main trial. In fact, OFDI-guided stent sizing even showed several positive aspects. The incidences of proximal stent-edge dissection with hematomas ($P = 0.04$) and irregular protrusions ($P = 0.014$) were significantly lower in the OFDI-guided PCI group than in the IVUS-guided PCI group. This might be because of the use of the gentle stent sizing strategy based on distal lumen measurement via OFDI. In this study, post-PCI OFDI showed a tendency toward a greater MSA in the IVUS-guided PCI group than in the OFDI-guided PCI group;

however, the follow-up minimal lumen area was comparable in both groups ($P = 0.18$) mainly owing to smaller neointimal proliferation (0.56 ± 0.30 mm^2 vs 0.80 ± 0.65 mm^2; $P = 0.057$) observed in the OFDI-guided PCI group. IVUS-guided PCI could account for increased neointimal hyperplasia due to more aggressive stent sizing compared with OFDI-guided PCI. In contrast, there was a significantly lower incidence of uncovered struts in the IVUS-guided PCI group than in the OFDI-guided PCI group, which might be a positive aspect of IVUS-guided PCI as compared with OFDI-guided PCI.

Optical coherence tomography-guided percutaneous coronary intervention in patients with acute coronary syndrome

It is well-known that ACS culprit lesions are different from those of chronic coronary syndrome (CCS) in terms of lipid-rich culprit plaques with or without TCFA and thrombus, which is more likely to induce no-reflow phenomenon. OCT has enabled an improved characterization of these culprit lesion features; thus, it is expected to be useful in this setting. Currently, there are only limited data regarding the impact of OCT guidance on PCI for patients with ACS. In the subgroup analysis of the CLI-OPCI II study,[18] Prati and colleagues[19] evaluated the prognostic impact of postprocedural culprit lesion OCT findings in patients with ACS undergoing PCI. They reported that suboptimal stent implantation, defined as the presence of significant residual intrastent plaque/thrombus protrusion (HR 2.35; $P < 0.01$), in-stent minimum lumen area <4.5 mm^2 (HR 2.72; $P < 0.01$), dissection >200 μm at the distal stent edge (HR 3.84; $P < 0.01$), and reference lumen area <4.5 mm^2 at either distal (HR 6.07; $P < 0.001$) or proximal (HR 8.50; $P < 0.001$) stent edges, were independently associated with device-oriented cardiovascular events. Postprocedural OCT assessment of the treated culprit lesion revealed at least one of these parameters in 55.2% of cases, along with an associated increased risk of device-oriented cardiovascular events during follow-up (17.9% vs 4.8%; $P < 0.001$). Both the presence of at least one of these parameters (HR 3.69; $P = 0.002$) and residual intrastent plaque/thrombus protrusion (HR 2.83; $P = 0.008$) were confirmed as independent predictors of device-oriented cardiovascular events. In this retrospective study of patients with ACS, a composite of OCT-defined suboptimal stent implantation characteristics at the culprit lesion and residual intrastent plaque/

thrombus protrusion was associated with adverse outcomes. Importantly, when compared with the CLI-OCPI II main study population that also included elective patients with stable coronary artery disease,[18] prevalence of the OCT-defined suboptimal stent deployment was significantly higher in patients with ACS (55.2% vs 31.0%; $P < 0.01$). These data indicate that patients with ACS are usually at increased risk of suboptimal stenting; hence, they might reap many benefits from OCT guidance when PCI is indicated.

DOCTORS (Does Optical Coherence Tomography Optimize Results of Stenting) was a multicenter, randomized trial comparing OCT-guided with angiography-guided PCI in 240 patients with non-ST-elevation ACS.[20] The primary endpoint of this study was the post-PCI fractional flow reserve (FFR) value. In the OCT group, stent sizing was performed according to the reference vessel size, and additional stent optimization was recommended if stent expansion (MSA/reference lumen area) was $\leq 80\%$. The OCT-guided group had a significantly higher post-PCI FFR (0.94 ± 0.04 vs 0.92 ± 0.05; $P = 0.005$) and prevalence of post-PCI FFR >0.9 (82.5% vs 64.2%; $P = 0.0001$) than the angiography-guided group, with significantly lower final angiographic diameter stenosis in the OCT-guided group than the angiography-guided group ($7.0 \pm 4.3\%$ vs $8.7 \pm 6.3\%$; $P = 0.01$, respectively). Additional stent optimization was conducted in 50% of cases in the OCT-guided group, while it was performed in 22.5% of cases in the angiography-guided group. After stent optimization, stent expansion increased from $78.9 \pm 12.4\%$ to $84.1 \pm 7.3\%$ in the OCT arm. Although these data imply the potential benefit of OCT-guided PCI in patients with ACS, no randomized study has evaluated the detailed impact of OCT-guided PCI on acute and chronic vessel reactions after stenting of ACS culprit lesions. Currently, the OPINION ACS study is ongoing and aims to clarify how IVUS and OFDI-guidance affect PCI with current-generation drug-eluting stents in patients with ACS,[21] and further evidence on these is anticipated.

TAKE-HOME MESSAGE

Several large-scale registries and randomized trials have shown the superiority of OCT to angiography and noninferiority to IVUS with respect to acute procedural and mid-term clinical outcomes. Although a dedicated randomized study comparing OCT-guided PCI with angiography-

Table 1
Clinical trials on optical coherence tomography versus intravascular ultrasound versus angiography-guided percutaneous coronary intervention

	Comparisons	Study Design	Study Subjects	Major Exclusion Criteria	Major Findings
Habara et al.[12]	OCT vs IVUS (n = 70)	Randomized: superiority of IVUS vs OCT	Stable angina (n = 63, 90%) and unstable angina (n = 7, 10%)	Patients with cardiogenic shock, left main coronary artery disease, totally occluded lesion, diffuse lesion (length >25 mm), bifurcation lesion, lesion of large vessel (reference vessel diameter >3.5 mm), lesion of severe tortuous vessel, serum creatinine >2 mg/dL	• Compared with IVUS guidance, OCT guidance was associated with smaller stent expansion and more frequent significant residual reference segment stenosis.
Jones et al.[11]	OCT vs IVUS vs angiography (n =)	Retrospective with adjustment with multivariate Cox analysis and propensity matching	Stable angina (n = 43,144, 57.1%) and ACS	Patients with acute ST-segment elevation myocardial infarction and patients undergoing pressure wire-guided PCI	• Improved long-term mortality (median of 4.8 years; interquartile range: 2.2 to 6.4 years) in OCT-guided PCI than angiography-guided PCI with no difference between OCT and IVUS guidance (HR: 0.88; 95% CI: 0.61 to 1.38; P = 0.43).
Iannaccone et al.[21]	OCT vs angiography (n = 540)	Retrospective propensity matching	ACS (UA: n = 88, 15%, NSTEMI: n = 192, 34% STEMI: n = 290, 51%)	N/A	• An OCT-guided approach reduced the number of stents used (primary endpoint). • The rates of MACE tended to be lower in the OCT-guided group (11% vs 16%; P = 0.06).
CLI-OPCI[10]	OCT vs angiography (n = 670)	Retrospective with multivariate analysis	Stable coronary artery disease (n = 264, 39%) NSTEMI (n = 197, 29%), STEMI (n = 209, 31%)	N/A	• OCT guidance was associated with a significantly lower risk of cardiac death or MI (odds ratio = 0.49 [0.25–0.96], P = 0.037).

Study	Comparison	Design	Population	Exclusion criteria	Results
Doctors[18]	OCT vs angiography (n = 240)	Randomized: superiority of OCT	NSTEMI (n = 240, 100%)	Patients with cardiogenic shock, severe renal insufficiency (estimated glomerular filtration rate (eGFR) $\leq$30 mL/min), left main disease; in-stent restenosis; presence of coronary artery bypass grafts; severely calcified or tortuous arteries; persistent ST-segment elevation	• Post-procedural FFR (primary endpoint) was significantly more improved with OCT guidance than with angiography guidance (0.94 $\pm$ 0.04 versus 0.92 $\pm$ 0.05, P = 0.005) • OCT guidance was associated with more frequent use of poststent balloon dilation than with angiography guidance (43% versus 12.5%, P < 0.0001), with lower residual stenosis (7.0 $\pm$ 4.3% versus 8.7 $\pm$ 6.3%, P = 0.01).
Sheth et al.[22]	OCT vs angiography (n = 642)	Retrospective with propensity matching	ST-segment-elevation myocardial infarction (n = 642, 100%)	Cardiogenic shock or known renal failure.	• OCT guidance was associated with a larger final in-stent minimum lumen diameter than with angiography guidance (2.99 $\pm$ 0.48 mm versus 2.79 $\pm$ 0.47 mm; P < 0.0001). • No significant difference in clinical outcomes at 1 year
OPINION[14]	OCT vs IVUS	Randomized: noninferiority of OCT vs IVUS	Stable angina (n = 715, 88%) Unstable angina (n = 101, 12%)	Patients with chronic kidney disease, cardiogenic shock, hemodialysis or peritoneal dialysis, triple-vessel disease, left main coronary artery disease, aorto-ostial lesion, chronic total occlusion,	• Target vessel failure occurred in 5.2% of patients undergoing OFDI-guided PCI, and 4.9% of patients undergoing IVUS-guided PCI, showing noninferiority of OFDI-

(continued on next page)

Table 1
(continued)

	Comparisons	Study Design	Study Subjects	Major Exclusion Criteria	Major Findings
				small vessel disease (reference vessel diameter <2.5 mm), coronary bypass graft, in-stent restenosis	guided PCI compared with IVUS-guided PCI (hazard ratio 1.07, upper limit of one-sided 95% confidence interval 1.80; $P_{noninferiority} = 0.042$). • The rate of binary restenosis was comparable between OFDI-guided PCI and IVUS-guided PCI (in-stent: 1.6% vs 1.6%, P = 1.00; and in-segment: 6.2% vs 6.0%, P = 1.00).
ILUMIEN III[13]	OCT vs IVUS vs angiography (n = 450)	Randomized: noninferiority of OCT vs IVUS, superiority of OCT vs angiography	Silent ischemia: (n = 133 29.6%, Stable angina: n = 153, 34%, Unstable angina: n = 85, 18.9%, NSTEMI: 63, 14%, Recent STEMI: n = 16, 3.6%)	Patients with cardiogenic shock, chronic kidney disease whose estimated creatinine clearance <30 mL/min, left main or ostial right coronary artery stenoses, bypass graft stenoses, chronic total occlusions, planned two-stent bifurcations, and in-stent restenosis.	• Regarding the final median minimum stent area, OCT guidance was noninferior to IVUS guidance (one-sided 97.5% lower CI −0.70 mm², P = 0.001), but not superior (P = 0.42). • OCT guidance was also not superior to angiography guidance (P = 0.12). • Procedural MACE was not statistically different among the groups.

Abbreviations: ACS, acute coronary syndrome; IVUS, intravascular ultrasound; MACE, major adverse cardiovascular events; NSTEMI, non-ST-elevation myocardial infarction; OCT, optical coherence tomography; STEMI, ST-elevation myocardial infarction.

guided PCI in terms of clinical outcomes is lacking, the aforementioned studies suggest that the superior clinical outcomes defined by randomized clinical trials on IVUS guidance in selected patients are likely applicable to OCT guidance. Indeed, a recent network meta-analysis including 17,882 patients who underwent angiography-, IVUS-, or OCT-guided implantation across 17 RCTs and 14 observational studies showed that IVUS or OCT guidance was associated with significant reductions in MACE and cardiovascular mortality as compared with angiographic guidance, without efficacy differences between IVUS and OCT.[22] However, strict inclusion and exclusion criteria have been set for each trial (Table 1). Regarding exclusion criteria, most of the studies excluded patients with cardiogenic shock, chronic renal failure, left main coronary artery disease, aorto-ostial lesion, chronic total occlusion, small vessel disease (reference vessel diameter <2.5 mm), coronary bypass graft, and in-stent restenosis. Thus, we need to pay careful attention when we try to apply this evidence to clinical practice. While there is strong evidence supporting the advantages of intravascular imaging to guide PCI in complex lesion morphology (long lesion and chronic total occlusion), there might be less benefit in simpler lesions or patients with more stable clinical presentations. Thus, the effects of routine use of intracoronary imaging guidance in an all-comers setting need to be established especially from the cost-benefit performance standpoint.

Furthermore, since intravascular imaging catheters such as IVUS and OCT are not magic wands, passing these modalities through the lesions cannot guarantee optimal stent expansion. The benefit from intravascular imaging guidance is clearly reliant on the image interpretation and subsequent reaction to optimize stenting. In this process, since stent sizing and post-stent procedure depend on the gauge (e.g., based on reference segment EEM vs lumen, proximal vs distal references or both, etc.), the procedures could vary even with the same modality used for PCI guidance. Indeed, the ILUMIEN III trial and OPINION study had similar concepts in comparing IVUS-guidance vs OCT-guidance, but different stent sizing protocols led to different acute procedural results. The ILUMIEN III trial showed similarities in MSA between OCT-guided PCI and IVUS-guided PCI, while smaller MSA was observed in the OFDI-guided PCI group than that in the IVUS-guided PCI group in the OPINION trial. Hence, the important thing is not whether one uses IVUS or OCT, but rather in the interpretation of the acquired image and translation into the subsequent procedures. Ideally, it is better to be aware of both stent sizing criteria and use them differently according to the lesion types (e.g., focal or diffuse, CCS or ACS, tapered or not tapered, etc.) to avoid periprocedural complications with an acceptable long-term prognosis. If there is a good command of using both criteria, OCT or IVUS might not be a big issue anymore.

CLINICS CARE POINTS

- Lipid plaque are considered potential risk factors for periprocedural complications of PCI.
- OCT could be a powerful tool to predict RA effect during PCI.
- While there is strong evidence supporting the advantages of intravascular imaging to guide PCI in complex lesion morphology (long lesion and chronic total occlusion), there might be less benefit in simpler lesions or patients with more stable clinical presentations.

DISCLOSURE

H. Otake received honoraria for lectures from Abbott Vascular ante Terumo Co.

REFERENCES

1. Kubo T, Akasaka T, Shite J, et al. OCT compared with IVUS in a coronary lesion assessment: the OPUS-CLASS study. JACC Cardiovasc Imaging 2013;6:1095–104.
2. Nishi T, Imura S, Kitahara H, et al. Head-to-head comparison of quantitative measurements between intravascular imaging systems: An in vitro phantom study. Int J Cardiol Heart Vasc 2021;36: 100867.
3. Garcia-Guimaraes M, Antuna P, De la Cuerda F, et al. High-definition IVUS versus OCT to assess coronary artery disease and results of stent implantation. JACC Cardiovasc Imaging 2020;13:519–21.
4. Yabushita H, Bouma BE, Houser SL, et al. Characterization of human atherosclerosis by optical coherence tomography. Circulation 2002;106: 1640–5.
5. Tanaka A, Imanishi T, Kitabata H, et al. Lipid-rich plaque and myocardial perfusion after successful

stenting in patients with non-ST-segment elevation acute coronary syndrome: an optical coherence tomography study. Eur Heart J 2009;30:1348–55.

6. Lee T, Yonetsu T, Koura K, et al. Impact of coronary plaque morphology assessed by optical coherence tomography on cardiac troponin elevation in patients with elective stent implantation. Circ Cardiovasc Interv 2011;4:378–86.

7. Ozaki Y, Tanaka A, Tanimoto T, et al. Thin-cap fibroatheroma as high-risk plaque for microvascular obstruction in patients with acute coronary syndrome. Circ Cardiovasc Imaging 2011;4:620–7.

8. Ino Y, Kubo T, Matsuo Y, et al. Optical coherence tomography predictors for edge restenosis after everolimus-eluting stent implantation. Circ Cardiovasc Interv 2016;9:e004231.

9. Kubo T, Shimamura K, Ino Y, et al. Superficial calcium fracture after PCI as assessed by OCT. JACC Cardiovasc Imaging 2015;8:1228–9.

10. Maejima N, Hibi K, Saka K, et al. Relationship between thickness of calcium on optical coherence tomography and crack formation after balloon dilatation in calcified plaque requiring rotational atherectomy. Circ J 2016;80:1413–9.

11. Tanimura K, Otake H, Kawamori H, et al. Prediction of the debulking effect of rotational atherectomy using optical frequency domain imaging. Heart Vessels 2021;36:1265–74.

12. Prati F, Di Vito L, Biondi-Zoccai G, et al. Angiography alone versus angiography plus optical coherence tomography to guide decision-making during percutaneous coronary intervention: the Centro per la Lotta contro l'Infarto-Optimisation of Percutaneous Coronary Intervention (CLI-OPCI) study. EuroIntervention 2012;8:823–9.

13. Jones DA, Rathod KS, Koganti S, et al. Angiography alone versus angiography plus optical coherence tomography to guide percutaneous coronary intervention: outcomes from the pan-London PCI cohort. JACC Cardiovasc Interv 2018;11:1313–21.

14. Habara M, Nasu K, Terashima M, et al. Impact of frequency-domain optical coherence tomography guidance for optimal coronary stent implantation in comparison with intravascular ultrasound guidance. Circ Cardiovasc Interv 2012;5:193–201.

15. Ali ZA, Maehara A, Genereux P, et al. Optical coherence tomography compared with intravascular ultrasound and with angiography to guide coronary stent implantation (ILUMIEN III: OPTIMIZE PCI): a randomised controlled trial. Lancet 2016;388:2618–28.

16. Kubo T, Shinke T, Okamura T, et al. Optical frequency domain imaging vs. intravascular ultrasound in percutaneous coronary intervention (OPINION trial): Study protocol for a randomized controlled trial. J Cardiol 2016;68:455–60.

17. Otake H, Kubo T, Takahashi H, et al. Optical frequency domain imaging versus intravascular ultrasound in percutaneous coronary intervention (OPINION Trial): Results from the OPINION Imaging Study. JACC Cardiovasc Imaging 2018;11:111–23.

18. Prati F, Romagnoli E, Burzotta F, et al. Clinical impact of OCT findings during PCI: the CLI-OPCI II Study. JACC Cardiovasc Imaging 2015;8:1297–305.

19. Prati F, Romagnoli E, Gatto L, et al. Clinical impact of suboptimal stenting and residual intrastent plaque/thrombus protrusion in patients with acute coronary syndrome: the CLI-OPCI ACS Substudy (Centro per la Lotta Contro L'Infarto-Optimization of Percutaneous Coronary Intervention in Acute Coronary Syndrome). Circ Cardiovasc Interv 2016; 9:e003726.

20. Meneveau N, Souteyrand G, Motreff P, et al. Optical coherence tomography to optimize results of percutaneous coronary intervention in patients with non-st-elevation acute coronary syndrome: results of the multicenter, randomized DOCTORS Study (Does Optical Coherence Tomography Optimize Results of Stenting). Circulation 2016;134:906–17.

21. Otake H, Kubo T, Shinke T, et al. OPtical frequency domain imaging vs. INtravascular ultrasound in percutaneous coronary InterventiON in patients with Acute Coronary Syndrome: study protocol for a randomized controlled trial. J Cardiol 2020; 76:317–21.

22. Buccheri S, Franchina G, Romano S, et al. Clinical outcomes following intravascular imaging-guided versus coronary angiography-guided percutaneous coronary intervention with stent implantation: a systematic review and Bayesian network meta-analysis of 31 studies and 17,882 patients. JACC Cardiovasc Interv 2017;10:2488–98.

OCT Emerging Technologies: Coronary Micro-optical Coherence Tomography

Kensuke Nishimiya, MD, PhD[a],
Radhika K. Poduval, PhD[b,c],
Guillermo J. Tearney, MD, PhD[b,c,d,e],*

KEYWORDS

- Optical coherence tomography (OCT) • Micro-OCT (µOCT) • Endothelial cells
- Inflammatory cells • Macrophage • Cholesterol crystals • Plaque erosion

KEY POINTS

- The resolution of commercially available optical coherence tomography (OCT) systems is in the range of 10 to 20 µm, which is insufficient to identify many key features of coronary lesions, such as the presence of neutrophils, macrophages, monocytes, vascular smooth muscle cells, and fibroblasts within the vessel wall.
- A new mode of OCT with approximately 1 to 2 µm spatial resolution, termed micro-OCT (µOCT), can visualize coronary microstructures at the cellular and subcellular levels in situ.
- A µOCT intravascular catheter has been developed for imaging in vivo and demonstrated in cadaver coronaries and animals in vivo.

INTRODUCTION

Intracoronary optical coherence tomography (OCT) plays an important role in interventional cardiology[1,2] by enabling visualization of accurate coronary morphology. The 10 to 20 µm spatial resolution of benchtop OCT[3,4] makes it possible to identify distinct architectural features of coronary plaques, such as macrophage accumulations,[5] calcific plates,[5–7] lipid,[5–7] thin fibrous caps,[1,5–8] cholesterol crystals,[6] and intimal/medial layer thickening,[7,9] information that has the potential to be clinically actionable.[10] Recent ISCHEMIA and REVIVED-BCIS2 trials[11,12] have highlighted the importance of optimal medical therapy (OMT) before an invasive strategy with percutaneous coronary intervention (PCI). To conduct cardiovascular disease risk stratification for OMT, it may be worthwhile to explore precursors of coronary atherosclerosis with a dedicated imaging tool. Clinically available OCT is less than adequate for this purpose because certain key features in these coronary lesions, such as neutrophils, macrophages, monocytes, vascular smooth muscle cells, and fibroblasts, are all below the resolution of these imaging systems. To bridge this gap, a new mode of OCT with approximately 1 to 2 µm spatial resolution, termed micro-OCT (µOCT), has been developed.[13] This review article summarizes the potential role of µOCT for

[a] Department of Cardiovascular Medicine, Tohoku University Graduate School of Medicine, 1-1 Seiryo-machi, Aoba-ku, Sendai, Miyagi, Japan; [b] Wellman Center for Photomedicine, Massachusetts General Hospital, Boston, MA, USA; [c] Harvard Medical School, Boston, MA, USA; [d] Department of Pathology, Massachusetts General Hospital, 55 Fruit Street, Boston, MA 02114, USA; [e] Harvard-MIT Division of Health Sciences and Technology Division, Cambridge, MA, USA
* Corresponding author. Department of Pathology, Harvard Medical School and Massachusetts General Hospital, Wellman Center for Photomedicine, 55 Fruit Street, Boston, MA 02114.
E-mail address: gtearney@partners.org

Intervent Cardiol Clin 12 (2023) 237–244
https://doi.org/10.1016/j.iccl.2023.01.001
2211-7458/23/© 2023 Elsevier Inc. All rights reserved.

visualizing coronary structures at cellular and sub-cellular levels, its potential clinical relevance, and future perspectives.

MICRO-OPTICAL COHERENCE TOMOGRAPHY
Development of Micro-optical Coherence Tomography

In 2011, µOCT imaging began as a bench-top microscopy system.[13] Further development of the technology resulted in a fiber-optic µOCT probe for luminal imaging.[14,15] In 2019, the fiber-optic imaging element was integrated into a catheter that was suitable for in vivo coronary imaging.[16] Results from µOCT imaging in animal models in vivo indicate the potential of this technology to be used in human subjects in the near future.[17]

Micro-optical Coherence Tomography for Identification of Coronary Endothelial Cells

The innermost layer of the coronary vessel wall, or intima, is covered entirely by a 1 to 2 µm-thick monolayer of endothelial cells (ECs) (Fig. 1). In en face scanning electron microscopy (SEM) images, a typical cobblestone pattern of coronary endothelial surface is apparent, which is termed "endothelial pavementing."[18] Disruption of the endothelial pattern and the EC barrier is thought to initiate coronary atherogenesis because it allows low-density lipoprotein and leukocytes to pass into the intima, leading to plaque formation.[19,20] Structural changes in the intima can be precipitated by local endothelial shear stress (ESS), which in turn accelerates endothelial dysfunction.[19] Previous studies have suggested that low or turbulent ESS changes the EC morphology away from the spindle-like shape aligned in the direction of flow.[21,22] Changes in the morphology of ECs are thought to have clinical significance, increasing vascular permeability,

and accelerating the formation of coronary plaque. Further loss of ECs can cause progressive plaque erosion that can lead to thrombotic lesions, one of the major histopathological precursors to acute coronary syndrome (ACS).[22–24] Therefore, visualizing ECs is a key step in understanding mechanisms behind human coronary plaque progression and disruption.

SEM is the current gold standard for endothelial imaging ex vivo.[18] However, SEM requires multiple steps of fixation, coating, dehydration, and desiccation to prepare the specimen. Unlike SEM, µOCT requires no sample preparation because it can be performed with fresh, unfixed tissue specimens.[13,25] Furthermore, an SEM image only affords a surface view. Thus, with SEM, it is difficult to correlate EC morphology with other coronary features beneath the endothelial surface. µOCT imaging is tomographic and can provide cross-sectional (see Fig. 1) and three-dimensional views (Fig. 2). Tomographic imaging allows visualization of microstructures within the inner layers of the coronary artery wall.[12,16,25,26] In a 3D-µOCT en face view of ex vivo coronary vessel wall, typical EC pavementing can be visualized, resembling the pattern seen by SEM imaging (see Fig. 2).[25] µOCT can also enable clear EC visualization in fresh swine coronary arteries ex vivo.[13] The accuracy of EC visualization with µOCT was validated statistically with SEM.[25] 3D-µOCT topological maps were generated from cross-sectional images containing depth information, which were referenced to the lumen-coronary interface, enabling the calculation of root mean squared error (RMSE)[27] as a measure of EC surface roughness. In a study by L Liu, and colleagues, the authors demonstrated a positive correlation between RMSE measured by 3D-µOCT to corresponding SEM images ($R^2 = 0.95$, $P = .01$),

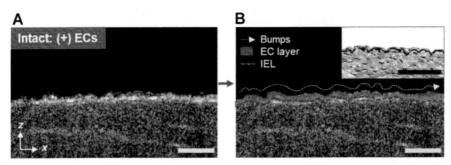

Fig. 1. (A) Cross-sectional µOCT image of a swine coronary artery ex vivo. (B) The same image as (A) with the endothelial cell layer morphology highlighted. Corresponding histology is shown in the inset. Coronary EC layer (blue area) forms bumps (yellow arrow) over the internal elastic lamina (IEL) (pink dashed line), which can be clearly visualized by µOCT. The appearance is similar to that seen by corresponding Movat's staining (small inset). Scale bars, 100 µm. (Unpublished data, obtained at the Massachusetts General Hospital.)

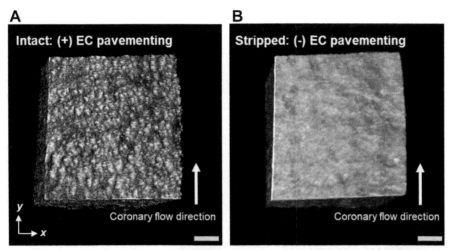

Fig. 2. En face view of 3D-μOCT images for coronary surface visualization in swine coronary artery ex vivo. (A) A representative image of 3D rendering of a μOCT dataset at the intact site of the coronary surface, showing the feature of "endothelial pavementing" and the direction of coronary flow (white arrow). (B) Coronary surface region showing a smooth surface but loss of endothelial features, suggestive of EC stripping within the IEL layer. Scale bars, 100 μm. (Figure and caption reprinted with permission from Nishimiya K, et al.[25])

indicating that surface-imaging with 3D-μOCT is statistically equivalent to the current gold standard SEM for the delineation of ECs.[13] Further evidence of the capacity of μOCT to image endothelial cells was demonstrated by stripping the endothelium from the top of swine coronary surface with biocompatible adhesives.[25] This experiment confirmed that a diminished surface roughness observed by 3D-μOCT of coronary indicates the denudation of ECs (see Fig. 2).[25] Identification of lesions with loss of ECs may be significant because it may provide a more precise means for locating erosive arterial regions with a propensity for thrombosis.

μOCT imaging of human cadaver coronaries revealed that unique patterns of ECs are linked to underlying coronary plaque morphology. For example, EC coverage was prominent over healthy coronary segments with intimal thickening, whereas EC coverage was lacking in lesions with superficial nodular calcification with a necrotic core (Fig. 3).[25] Further, human ECs over fibroatheromatous plaque were sparse relative to those over a healthy coronary segment (see Fig. 3).[25] RMSE and surface roughness were significantly decreased in fibroatheromatous and fibrocalcific plaques compared with less severe atherosclerotic lesions (see Fig. 3). It has also been reported that apoptotic macrophages are not efficiently cleared by efferocytosis in thin-cap fibroatheroma (TCFA) lesions.[28] This can make TCFAs vulnerable to secondary necrosis, with progressive enlargement of the necrotic core and its fibrous cap thinning.[29]

Therefore, intimal surface roughness measurement through μOCT imaging (expressed as RMSE) could be a novel marker of early manifestation of coronary atherosclerosis and may also be helpful to establish a more precise quantification of plaque vulnerability in humans.

Micro-optical Coherence Tomography for Identification of Inflammatory Cells

Studies have suggested that a therapeutic strategy targeting macrophage inflammasome-generated vascular inflammation (colchicine and an anti-IL1β-mab) decreases residual risk of coronary artery disease.[30–32] Additionally, neutrophil adhesion to the coronary endothelial surface and subsequent monocyte/macrophage infiltration plays a key role in developing coronary atherosclerotic lesions.[33] Inflammasome activation (NLRP3 gene) in macrophages accelerates the process of inflammatory cytokine/chemokine production and activation.[34] Recently, attention has been directed toward the role of neutrophils expelling neutrophil extracellular traps (NETs) as a phenomenon that can exacerbate the inflammasome-generated vascular inflammation.[35] μOCT has the potential to highlight some of these findings, given its capability to enable the visualization of specific inflammatory cells ex vivo in human coronaries.[13,26] Monocytes can be seen by μOCT, seen as large cells with scant cytoplasm and bean-shaped nuclei adhering to the intimal surface (Fig. 4A).[13] Macrophages present in μOCT as large, round or ellipsoidal cells that are highly scattering and

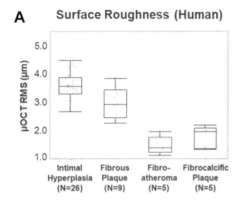

A Surface Roughness (Human)

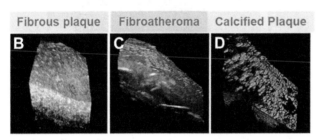

Fibrous plaque | Fibroatheroma | Calcified Plaque

μOCT Images of Human Cadaver Coronary Arteries

Fig. 3. Endothelial surface roughness measurement results and representative μOCT images for varying plaque morphologies. (A) Bar graph showing RMSE calculation measured by μOCT for different coronary lesions. RMSE was lowest for fibroatheroma. Statistically significant differences were found between intimal hyperplasia vs fibrous/fibrocalcific plaques and in fibrous plaques vs fibroatheroma/fibrocalcific plaques. Statistical differences were examined using one-way analysis of variance and post hoc analysis with the Tukey's test. (B–D) Representative μOCT images for varying plaque morphologies. Compared with intimal hyperplasia (B), ECs over fibroatheroma and fibrocalcific plaques are sparse (C, D). (Figure and caption reprinted with permission from Nishimiya K, et al.[25])

flocculent. This finding was supported by conducting μOCT of cultured macrophages in vitro.[26] It was also observed that phagocytosis of cholesterol crystals exhibited elevated cytoplasmic scattering in μOCT images, relative to those with an absence of cholesterol crystals.[26] 3D-μOCT grants the capacity of clear delineation of individual macrophages phagocytosing highly scattering cholesterol crystals (Fig. 4B, C).[26] Moreover, leukocytes adhering to the coronary endothelial surface have also been imaged by μOCT (Fig. 5A–C).[26] Pseudopods of these inflammatory cells highlight anchor sites to the endothelium (Fig. 5D). While not yet demonstrated, μOCT technology has the resolution to identify

neutrophils with NETs that are likely to induce ECs apoptosis and result in coronary plaque erosion.[36]

Intravascular Micro-optical Coherence Tomography

Recently, intravascular μOCT catheters were fabricated and used to conduct imaging of human cadaver coronary arteries and imaging of atherosclerotic rabbit aortae in vivo.[16] μOCT circumferential views were able to display vascular smooth muscle cells in human cadaver coronary lesions with intimal thickening and cholesterol crystal accumulation in human fibroatheromatous plaques ex vivo (Fig. 6).[16] Further,

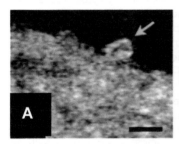
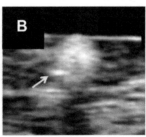
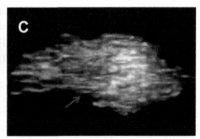

Fig. 4. μOCT for visualization of monocytes and macrophages. (A) Monocytes can be seen by μOCT, visualized as large cells with scant cytoplasm and bean-shaped nuclei adhering to the intimal surface (green arrow). (B, C) Representative 2D μOCT and 3D-μOCT images of a macrophage within a cadaver human coronary artery. A scattering cholesterol inclusion is present within the cytoplasm, indicating phagocytosis (yellow arrow in B; red in C). Scale bars, 30 μm for (A). (Figure and caption reprinted with permission from Kashiwagi M, et al.[26])

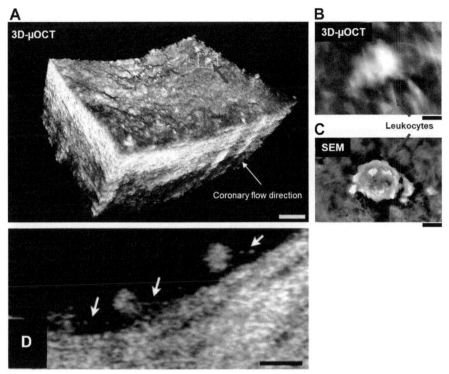

Fig. 5. 3D-μOCT image depicting leukocytes' adhering to the coronary luminal surface. (A) 3D-μOCT of EC morphology of a lipid-rich human coronary plaque with adhered leukocytes (*red arrows* in A, B). (C) Coregistered SEM image showing an individual leukocyte tethered to the surface. (D) Pseudopods of these inflammatory cells highlight anchor sites to the endothelium Scale bars for A, 100 μm; B and C, 10 μm; D, 30 μm. (*white arrows*) indicates the direction of coronary flow. ([A–C] *Unpublished data*, obtained at the Massachusetts General Hospital. [D] Figure and caption reprinted with permission from Liu L, et al.[13])

cross-sectional μOCT images obtained with this catheter exhibited macrophage diapedesis in early coronary lesions ex vivo. 3D-μOCT images allowed clear delineation of individual macrophages transmigrating through the endothelium (Fig. 7A, B) toward an intimal cholesterol crystal deposit (Fig. 7C) or with opposing pseudopodia in a "kissing" configuration (Fig. 7D).[16]

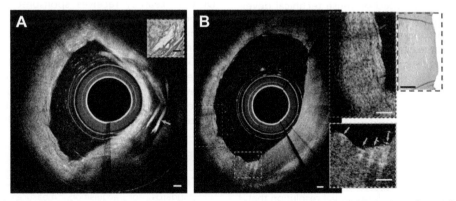

Fig. 6. Catheter-based intravascular μOCT of a human cadaver coronary ex vivo. (A) A circumferential view of μOCT clearly showing multiple cholesterol crystals characterized by reflections from their top and bottom surfaces (*blue arrows*). (B) A cross-section of an artery exhibiting probable smooth muscle cells (*red arrows* in the inset with matching histology) and macrophages undergoing diapedesis (*green arrows* in the *inset*). Scale bars, 100 μm. (Figure and capture reprinted with permission from Yin B, et al.[16])

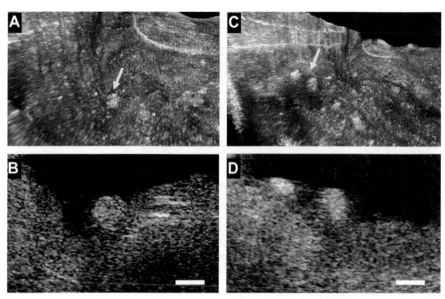

Fig. 7. Intravascular μOCT of macrophages in a human cadaver coronary artery ex vivo. (A) Individual macrophages (*yellow arrows*) residing on the surface of a fibroatheromatous plaque that (B) seemed to be transmigrating through the endothelium toward a deposit of intimal cholesterol crystals. (C) 3D-μOCT image showing a pair of macrophages tethered to the surface, (D) polarized toward one another with extended pseudopodia. Scale bars, 50 μm. (Reprinted with permission from Yin B, Hyun C, Gardecki JA, Tearney GJ. Extended depth of focus for coherence-based cellular imaging. Optica. 2017;4(8):959-965. © The Optical Society.)

SUMMARY

μOCT offers an enhancement of axial and lateral resolution by an order of magnitude compared with commercially available OCT. Ongoing studies demonstrate the ability of μOCT to visualize key cellular and subcellular features involved in coronary atherogenesis and progression. For example, catheter-based μOCT imaging has shown its potential to display individual crystals and inflammatory cells not only in human coronary plaques ex vivo but also in animal models in vivo. Based on these technical developments and results, μOCT is a promising next-generation imaging technology for improving the clinical understanding of coronary artery disease and for potentially guiding individualized treatment based on the predictive capacity of cellular and subcellular plaque morphology.

CLINICS CARE POINTS

- μOCT offers 1 to 2 μm spatial resolution that is anrepresents more than an order magnitude improvement over current clinical OCT systems.
- μOCT enables clear visualization of endothelial cells, neutrophils, macrophages,

individual crystals, monocytes, and vascular smooth muscle cells, which are relevant for the study of the pathogenesis and progression of coronary atherosclerosis.

- In the future, catheter-based μOCT may be helpful for the detailed prediction of coronary atherosclerosis progression in living patients in vivo.

DISCLOSURES

Dr G.J. Tearney receives sponsored research support from Canon, Japan and Verdure Biotech Holdings. He also has a financial/fiduciary interest in SpectraWave, a company developing an OCT-NIRS intracoronary imaging system and catheter. His financial/fiduciary interest was reviewed and is managed by the Massachusetts General Hospital and MGB HealthCare in accordance with their conflict-of-interest policies.

REFERENCES

1. Tearney GJ, Regar E, Akasaka T, et al. Consensus standards for acquisition, measurement, and reporting of intravascular optical coherence tomography studies: a report from the International Working Group for Intravascular Optical Coherence Tomography Standardization and Validation. J Am Coll Cardiol 2012;59(12):1058–72.

2. Ali ZA, Karimi Galougahi K, Mintz GS, et al. Intra-coronary optical coherence tomography: state of the art and future directions. EuroIntervention 2021;17(2):e105–23.

3. Tearney GJ, Brezinski ME, Bouma BE, et al. In vivo endoscopic optical biopsy with optical coherence tomography. Science (1979) 1997; 276(5321):2037–9.

4. Yun SH, Tearney GJ, Vakoc BJ, et al. Comprehensive volumetric optical microscopy in vivo. Nat Med 2006;12(12):1429–33.

5. Tearney GJ, Yabushita H, Houser SL, et al. Quantification of macrophage content in atherosclerotic plaques by optical coherence tomography. Circulation 2003;107(1):113–9.

6. Tearney GJ, Waxman S, Shishkov M, et al. Three-dimensional coronary artery microscopy by intra-coronary optical frequency domain imaging. JACC Cardiovasc Imaging 2008;1(6):752–61.

7. Kume T, Akasaka T, Kawamoto T, et al. Assessment of coronary intima-media thickness by optical coherence tomography comparison with intravascular ultrasound. Circ J 2005;69(8):903–7.

8. Yabushita H, Bouma BE, Houser SL, et al. Characterization of human atherosclerosis by optical coherence tomography. Circulation 2002;106(13): 1640–5.

9. Gerbaud E, Weisz G, Tanaka A, et al. Multi-laboratory inter-institute reproducibility study of IVOCT and IVUS assessments using published consensus document definitions. European Heart Journal-Cardiovascular Imaging 2016;17(7):756–64.

10. Araki M, Park SJ, Dauerman HL, et al. Optical coherence tomography in coronary atherosclerosis assessment and intervention. Nat Rev Cardiol 2022; 19(10):684–703.

11. Maron DJ, Hochman JS, Reynolds HR, et al. Initial invasive or conservative strategy for stable coronary disease. N Engl J Med 2020;382(15):1395–407.

12. Perera D, Clayton T, O'Kane PD, et al. Percutaneous revascularization for ischemic left ventricular dysfunction. N Engl J Med 2022;387(15):1351–60.

13. Liu L, Gardecki JA, Nadkarni SK, et al. Imaging the subcellular structure of human coronary atherosclerosis using micro–optical coherence tomography. Nat Med 2011;17(8):1010–4.

14. Yin B, Chu KK, Liang CP, et al. μOCT imaging using depth of focus extension by self-imaging wavefront division in a common-path fiber optic probe. Opt Express 2016;24(5):5555–64.

15. Yin B, Hyun C, Gardecki JA, et al. Extended depth of focus for coherence-based cellular imaging. Optica 2017;4(8):959–65.

16. Yin B, Piao Z, Nishimiya K, et al. 3D cellular-resolution imaging in arteries using few-mode interferometry. Light Sci Appl 2019;8(1):1–9.

17. Nishimiya K, Tearney G. Micro Optical Coherence Tomography for Coronary Imaging. Front Cardiovasc Med 2021;8:613400.

18. Pasternak RC, Baughman KL, Fallon JT, et al. Scanning electron microscopy after coronary transluminal angioplasty of normal canine coronary arteries. Am J Cardiol 1980;45(3):591–8.

19. Aird WC. Vascular bed-specific thrombosis. J Thromb Haemostasis 2007;5:283–91.

20. Vanhoutte PM, Shimokawa H, Feletou M, et al. Endothelial dysfunction and vascular disease–a 30th anniversary update. Acta Physiol 2017;219(1): 22–96.

21. Malek AM, Alper SL, Izumo S. Hemodynamic Shear Stress and Its Role in Atherosclerosis. JAMA 1999; 282(21):2035–42.

22. Farb A, Burke AP, Tang AL, et al. Coronary plaque erosion without rupture into a lipid core: a frequent cause of coronary thrombosis in sudden coronary death. Circulation 1996;93(7):1354–63.

23. Jia H, Abtahian F, Aguirre AD, et al. In vivo diagnosis of plaque erosion and calcified nodule in patients with acute coronary syndrome by intravascular optical coherence tomography. J Am Coll Cardiol 2013;62(19):1748–58.

24. Otsuka F, Joner M, Prati F, et al. Clinical classification of plaque morphology in coronary disease. Nat Rev Cardiol 2014;11(7):379–89.

25. Nishimiya K, Yin B, Piao Z, et al. Micro-optical coherence tomography for endothelial cell visualization in the coronary arteries. JACC Cardiovasc Imaging 2019;12(9):1878–80.

26. Kashiwagi M, Liu L, Chu KK, et al. Feasibility of the assessment of cholesterol crystals in human macrophages using micro optical coherence tomography. PLoS One 2014;9(7):e102669.

27. Castellino M, Stolojan V, Virga A, et al. Chemico-physical characterisation and in vivo biocompatibility assessment of DLC-coated coronary stents. Anal Bioanal Chem 2013;405(1):321–9.

28. Kojima Y, Weissman IL, Leeper NJ. The role of efferocytosis in atherosclerosis. Circulation 2017; 135(5):476–89.

29. Tabas I. Macrophage death and defective inflammation resolution in atherosclerosis. Nat Rev Immunol 2010;10(1):36–46.

30. Everett BM, Thuren T, MacFadyen JG, et al. Antiinflammatory Therapy with Canakinumab for Atherosclerotic Disease. N Engl J Med 2017;377(12):1119–31.

31. Tardif JC, Kouz S, Waters DD, et al. Efficacy and safety of low-dose colchicine after myocardial infarction. N Engl J Med 2019;381(26):2497–505.

32. Nidorf SM, Fiolet ATL, Mosterd A, et al. Colchicine in patients with chronic coronary disease. N Engl J Med 2020;383(19):1838–47.

33. Libby P. The changing landscape of atherosclerosis. Nature 2021;592(7855):524–33.

34. Grebe A, Hoss F, Latz E. NLRP3 inflammasome and the IL-1 pathway in atherosclerosis. Circ Res 2018;122(12):1722–40.

35. Warnatsch A, Ioannou M, Wang Q, et al. Neutrophil extracellular traps license macrophages for cytokine production in atherosclerosis. Science (1979) 2015;349(6245):316–20.

36. Quillard T, Araújo HA, Franck G, et al. TLR2 and neutrophils potentiate endothelial stress, apoptosis and detachment: implications for superficial erosion. Eur Heart J 2015;36(22):1394–404.

The Ability of Near-Infrared Spectroscopy to Identify Vulnerable Patients and Plaques: A Systematic Review and Meta-Analysis

Ronald D. Bass, BA[a], Joseph Phillips, BS, MS[b],
Jorge Sanz Sánchez, MD, PhD[c,d], Priti Shah, MSc[e],
Stephen Sum, PhD[e], Ron Waksman, MD[f],
Hector M. Garcia-Garcia, MD, PhD[f,*]

KEYWORDS

- NIRS • Vulnerable plaque • ACS • LRP

KEY POINTS

- A near-infrared spectroscopy (NIRS) meta-analysis provides a more precise estimate of the efficacy of NIRS.
- NIRS-derived lipid core burden index (LCBI) is an effective method for quantifying and identifying high-risk plaques and patients at increased risk of future MACE/MACCE.
- A maxLCBI$_{4mm}$ of 400 or greater seems to be an effective threshold for classifying at-risk plaques.

INTRODUCTION

Coronary artery disease continues to be a major cause of global morbidity and mortality despite medical advancements and effective preventive measures.[1] Acute coronary syndromes (ACS) are most often caused by rupture or fissure of a lipid-rich core-containing plaque and a large plaque burden, termed a vulnerable plaque.[2,3] Autopsy findings determined that these atheromas have a large plaque size, cholesterol-rich lipid core, and thin fibrous cap.[4] Atheromas tend to occur at multiple sites resulting in high atherosclerotic burden, which confers to a patient at high-risk of adverse cardiac events.[2] More recently, research has focused on preemptively identifying at-risk plaques and patients in a more proactive strategy of targeted secondary prevention.

Currently, the only imaging modality validated to identify lipid-rich plaques is near-infrared spectroscopy (NIRS).[5] NIRS uses unique technology via an add-on optic fiber as part of an imaging system attached to an intravascular ultrasound (IVUS) catheter that can easily identify lipid-rich plaque.[5] NIRS is able to deliver quantitative data regarding lipid composition within coronary artery walls, providing a more precise identification of vulnerable plaques than previously available,[6] which may provide clinicians with improved patient-level risk estimation for more targeted interventions.

---

[a] School of Medicine, Georgetown University, 3800 Reservoir Road, NorthWest, Washington, DC 20007, USA; [b] University of Iowa Hospitals and Clinics, 200 Hawkins Drive Iowa City, IA 52242, USA; [c] Hospital Universitari I Politecnic La Fe, Avinguda de Fernando Abril Martorell, no 106, 46026 València, Spain; [d] Centro de Investigación Biomedica en Red (CIBERCV), Avenue, Monforte de Lemos, 3-5. Pabellón 11. Planta 0. 28029 Madrid, Spain; [e] InfraRedx, A Nipro Company, 28 Crosby Drive, Suite 100, Bedford, MA 01730, USA; [f] Interventional Cardiology, MedStar Washington Hospital Center, 110 Irving Street, Suite 4B-1, Washington, DC, 20010, USA
* Corresponding author. 110 Irving Street, Suite 4B-1, Washington, DC, 20010,
E-mail addresses: hector.m.garciagarcia@medstar.net; hect2701@gmail.com

Intervent Cardiol Clin 12 (2023) 245–256
https://doi.org/10.1016/j.iccl.2022.10.006
2211-7458/23/© 2022 Elsevier Inc. All rights reserved.

Although NIRS has been evaluated in the context of many different clinical scenarios, for the purposes of this study, we chose to focus on the association of NIRS and cardiovascular (CV) outcomes. Emerging evidence suggest that NIRS-derived lipid core burden index (LCBI) provides prognostic data at the patient level as well as the plaque level. Individual studies evaluating the role of NIRS are characterized by the inclusion of a small number of patients and may not provide adequately powered analysis, thus prompting the need for a systematic appraisal of treatment effects and quality of evidence. Therefore, this systematic review and meta-analysis aims to compile the currently available data regarding the prognostic value of NIRS-derived LCBI on adverse cardiac outcomes to provide more precise effect estimates.

METHODS
Protocol
This systematic review and meta-analysis was performed according to the Preferred Reporting Items for Systematic Reviews and Meta-Analyses (PRISMA) reporting guidelines.[7] The corresponding author had full access to all the data and had final responsibility for the decision to submit for publication. The data supporting the findings in this study are available from the corresponding author on reasonable request.

Search Strategy
We performed a comprehensive literature search of all published studies—retrospective, prospective, observational—available through PubMed and Ovid (inception through December 31, 2021), without language restrictions. Case reports, letters to the editor, reviews, and book chapters were not included in this meta-analysis. Key search terms used were, "NIRS," "IVUS," "LCBI," "MACE," "MACCE," "coronary artery disease," "coronary heart disease," "angina," "myocardial infarction," "acute myocardial infarct," "myocardial ischemia," "acute coronary syndrome," "ischemic heart disease" including their subheadings, MeSH terms, and all synonyms. References for each of the studies selected were also screened. The PRISMA guidelines were applied for this search process.

Selection Criteria
Studies were eligible if they met the following criteria: (1) investigated the diagnostic performance of NIRS in predicting adverse cardiac outcomes; (2) in a patient population undergoing an invasive catheterization laboratory procedure, regardless of indication; (3) involving a

unique patient population not included in another study; and (4) reported at least 1 of the following CV outcomes: all-cause mortality, CV mortality, myocardial infarction, stroke, or urgent coronary revascularization. Study selection was performed by 2 independent reviewers (R.B. and J.P.), first by screening of titles and abstracts, followed by review of full texts and their corresponding references. In cases in which there was a disagreement over eligibility, a third reviewer (H.G.) assessed the discrepancy, and decisions were reached by consensus. Quality of the data was analyzed using the Downs and Black Checklist or the Cochrane Risk of Bias tools, as applicable, by study type. An overview of referenced studies is provided in Table 1.

Data Extraction
Data on study characteristics, patient characteristics, and endpoint event rates were independently extracted and organized into a structured data set by 2 reviewers (R.B. and J.P.), compared, and reported in Table 2. Any discrepancy resulted in reevaluation of the primary data and involvement of a third reviewer (H.G.), with disagreements resolved by consensus.

Outcomes of Interest
The central illustration (Fig. 1) shows an example of a NIRS-derived chemogram and the value of NIRS in identifying high-risk patients and plaques. The prespecified primary endpoint in this study was major adverse cardiovascular and cerebrovascular events (MACCE). For trials not reporting MACCE, MACE was chosen as primary endpoint.[8–14] Note that maxLCBI$_{4mm}$ was used in all studies except Danek and colleagues, which did not have the data available, and therefore used the LCBI of the vessel with highest lipid burden.[10] Thus, the authors of this article use the term LCBI to refer to all the NIRS-derived measurements for purposes of the primary analysis. Note that the maxLCBI$_{4mm}$ refers to the 4 mm long segment with the maximum LCBI. The authors of this study then investigated their own secondary endpoint using a threshold maxLCBI$_{4mm}$ at or around 400 as suggested by prior studies including Waksman and colleagues.[13] Each endpoint was assessed according to the definitions reported in the original study protocols. The list of endpoints for each study is listed in Table 3 along with the definitions of each endpoint.

Risk of Bias
Methodological quality of included studies was assessed using the Risk of Bias In Nonrandomized Studies of Interventions assessment Tool from Cochrane handbook (ROBINS-I). Two

Table 1
Study overviews

Trial/Author Year	Study Design	Multicenter	Population	Follow-Up
Oemrawsingh, et al,[8] 2014	Observational (prospective) Primary endpoint: MACCE	No	Patients with clinical indication for diagnostic coronary angiography and/or PCI due to ACS or stable CAD	1 y
Madder, et al,[9] 2016	Observational (prospective) Primary endpoint: MACCE	No	Patients with clinical indication for invasive coronary angiography and/or PCI due to ACS or stable CAD	1.7 y ± 0.4 y
Danek, et al,[10] 2017	Observational (prospective) Primary endpoint: MACE	No	Patients with clinically indicated cardiac catheterization and NIRS imaging due to ACS or stable CAD	Median 5.3 y
Schuurman, et al,[11] 2017	Observational (prospective) Primary endpoint: MACE	No	Patients undergoing diagnostic coronary angiography or PCI due to ACS or stable CAD	Median 4.1 y
Karlsson, et al,[12] 2019	Observational (retrospective enrollment, prospective follow-up) Primary endpoint: MACCE	Yes	Patients with clinical indication for coronary catheterization due to ACS or stable CAD	Mean 2.9 ± 1.3 y
LRP Study Waksman, et al,[13] 2019	Prospective, cohort Primary endpoint: MACE	Yes	Patients with indication for cardiac catheterization with possible ad hoc PCI due to known or suspected ACS or stable CAD	2 y
PROSPECT II Erlinge, et al,[14] 2021	Prospective, observational Primary endpoint: MACE	Yes	Patients intended for coronary angiography ± PCI due to recent STEMI or NSTEMI enrolled after successful intervention of all flow-limiting culprit lesions	Median 3.7 y

Abbreviations: CAD, coronary artery disease; NSTEMI, non-ST segment elevation myocardial infarction; PCI, percutaneous coronary intervention; STEMI, ST segment elevation myocardial infarction.

investigators (R.B. and J.P) independently assessed 7 domains of bias: (1) confounding, (2) selection of participants, (3) classification of interventions, (4) deviations from intended interventions, (5) missing outcome data, (6) measurement of the outcome, and (7) selection of the reported results.

Statistical Analysis
Odds ratios (OR) and 95% confidence intervals (CI) were calculated using the DerSimonian and Laird random-effects model, with the estimate of heterogeneity being taken from the Mantel-Haenszel method. When the required numbers to pool the data were not available in the text

Table 2
Background characteristics

Trial/Author	Age[b] (y)	Men (%)	HTN (%)	DM2 (%)	HLD (%)	Prior MI (%)	Prior PCI (%)	Prior CABG (%)	Prior Stroke (%)	Index Presentation (%)
Oemrawsingh, et al,[8] 2014	63.4	72.9	56.2	20.2	56.7	38.9	38.4	3.0	3.0	Composite ACS 46.8 Stable Symptoms 53.2
Madder, et al,[9] 2016	62.5	68.6	57.9	19.8	57.9	14.0	18.2	NR	5.0	Composite ACS 85.1 Stable Symptoms 14.9
Danek, et al,[10] 2017[a]	63.5	99	95	50	93	36	11	23	11.0	Composite ACS 39 Stable Symptoms 61
Schuurman, et al,[11] 2017	62.5	76.7	60.0	21.5	57.5	34.2	35.6	2.2	5.8	Composite ACS 42.5 Stable Symptoms 57.5
Karlsson, et al,[12] 2019	66.5	70.8	53.5	19.4	NR	29.2	NR	NR	9.7	Composite ACS 81.9 Stable Symptoms 18.1
LRP Study (Waksman, et al,[13] 2019)	64.0	69.5	80.4	36.7	80.3	23.5	44.9	NR	NR	Composite ACS 53.7 Stable Symptoms 46.3
PROSPECT II (Erlinge, et al,[14] 2021)	63.0	83.0	37.2[c]	12.1	25.2[d]	9.9	11.9	0.0	5.2	Composite ACS 100.0

Included background characteristics refer to the full study populations as defined in Table 1 of the individual studies.

Abbreviations: CABG, coronary artery bypass graft; CAD, coronary artery disease; DM2, diabetes mellitus type 2; HLD, hyperlipidemia; HTN, hypertension; MI, myocardial infarction; NSTEMI, non-ST segment elevation MI; PCI, percutaneous coronary intervention; SAP, stable angina pectoris; STEMI, ST segment elevation MI; Sx, symptoms; UAP, unstable angina pectoris.

[a] Authors did not present any decimals.
[b] All ages are reported as means except Erlinge et al. is a median.
[c] HTN in PROSPECT-II defined as hypertension requiring medication.
[d] HLD in PROSPECT-II defined as hyperlipidemia requiring medication.

or tables, we used an online semiautomated software to extract underlying numerical data from applicable Kaplan-Meier curves provided to determine the number of events above and below the relevant LCBI threshold in each study (WebPlotDigitizer 4.5, Ankit Rohatgi, Pacifica, California, USA). The presence of heterogeneity among studies was evaluated with the Cochran Q chi-square test, with $P \leq .10$ considered of statistical significance, and using the I^2 test to evaluate inconsistency. A value of 0% indicates no observed heterogeneity, and larger values indicate increasing heterogeneity. I^2 values of 25% or lesser, 50% or lesser, and greater than 50% indicated low, moderate, and high heterogeneity, respectively. A prespecified sensitivity analyses

was performed by removing the studies not using a threshold maxLCBI$_{4mm}$ at or around 400.

Analyses were performed according to the intention-to-treat principle. The statistical level of significance was 2-tailed $P < .05$. Statistical analyses were performed with the Stata software version 13.1 (StataCorp LP, College Station, Texas, USA).

RESULTS
Search Results
A total of 7 studies involving 2948 patients were identified for this study as shown in Table 1. Each study was published within the last 10 years. All were observational studies with prospective follow-up.

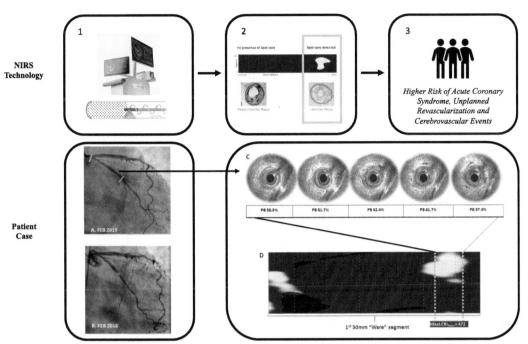

Fig. 1. The near-infrared spectroscopy instrument and example patient case. The top half of the image contains 3 panels, labeled 1 to 3 and outlined with black boxes, to introduce the near-infrared spectroscopy technology. The top image in panel 1 shows the NIRS machine while the bottom image in panel 1 shows the Dualpro catheter that delivers light to the vessel wall. Panel 2 is an example chemogram derived from the machine in panel 1. The red and yellow colors differentiate plaque characteristics. Yellow color on the chemogram as shown represents lipid core plaque. There is a yellow box around the identified lipid core plaque. Panel 3 emphasizes the association of this type of lipid core plaque with patient morbidity and mortality, particularly events defined in MACE/MACCE such as acute coronary syndrome, unplanned coronary revascularization, and cerebrovascular events. The bottom half of the figure shows a patient case representing the utility of NIRS.[13] There are 2 parts outlined with black boxes, each with 2 panels, labeled (A–D). Panel A shows the baseline coronary angiography of the left circumflex artery with no stenosis at the time of study enrollment. The light blue lines correspond to the 30 mm Ware segment as defined in the study protocol. Panel B shows the follow-up coronary angiography 1 year later, this time with a new significant lesion on the left circumflex. The intravascular ultrasound grayscale images in Panel C correspond to the maxLCBI$_{4mm}$ at baseline. The plaque burden of each 1-mm interval frame is found underneath each intravascular ultrasound image. In each interval, the plaque burden is moderate, between 57.4% and 62.4%. (A) NIRS-derived chemogram of the 30 mm Ware segment at baseline is seen in Panel D, indicating a maxLCBI$_{4mm}$ of 472. This patient case emphasizes the importance of NIRS-identification of lipid-rich plaque. Even though the angiography at baseline showed no stenosis, the area with maxLCBI$_{4mm}$ as discovered by NIRS was the culprit of a new lesion 1 year later. NIRS can predict potential areas of complication and provide an opportunity for prevention at the patient and plaque level.

Two of the studies, Schuurman and colleagues and Oemrawsingh and colleagues, included the same study population with results reported at different periods of follow-up.[8,11] Because Schuurman and colleagues published results with a greater duration of follow-up and larger sample size the authors chose to include those results and exclude Oemrawsingh and colleagues from the statistical analysis. Furthermore, although the total study population in Danek and colleagues was 239 patients, available data for nontarget vessel LCBI was only available for 39 patients.

Baseline Characteristics

Main baseline characteristics of included patients for each individual study are summarized in Table 2. Most patients were men with a mean age ranging from 62.5 to 66.5 years. The percentage of patients with hypertension ranged between 37.2% and 95%, whereas those with type 2 diabetes ranged from 12.1% to 50%. The presence of hyperlipidemia was between 25.2% and 93%. A subset of patients in each study experienced prior myocardial infarction, ranging from 9.9% to 38.9% of the populations. ACS was the index presentation in between 39% and 100% of patients.

Table 3
Outcome definitions

Trial/Author	MACCE	MACE	ACS	Cerebrovascular Events	MI	Unstable Angina	Unplanned Coronary Revascularization	Cardiac Death
Oemrawsingh, et al,[8] 2014	All-cause mortality Nonfatal ACS Stroke Unplanned coronary revascularization	NR	Per guidelines of the European Society of Cardiology	Per guidelines of the European Stroke Organization	NR	NR	PCI or CABG which initially was not planned after index angiography and study enrollment	NR
Madder, et al,[9] 2016	All-cause mortality Nonfatal ACS Acute cerebrovascular events	NR	MI or UA arising from a de novo culprit lesion and requiring revascularization	TIA or stroke	Universal definition	ACS presentations in the absence of cardiac biomarker elevations	NR	NR
Danek, et al,[10] 2017	NR	Cardiac death ACS Unplanned coronary revascularization Stroke after discharge from index hospitalization	Third Universal Definition of Myocardial Infarction	NR	Third Universal Definition	Third Universal Definition	PCI or CABG that was not planned after the index coronary angiography and NIRS imaging procedure	NR
Schuurman, et al,[11] 2017	NR	All-cause death Non-fatal ACS Unplanned coronary revascularization	Per guidelines of the European Society of Cardiology	NR TIA or stroke	ESC Guidelines NR	ESC Guidelines NR	Any PCI or CABG that was not planned after the index angiography and enrollment in the study NR	Any death due to proximate cardiac cause, unwitnessed death or death of unknown cause NR

	All-cause mortality Recurrent ACS requiring revascularization Cerebrovascular events	Event requiring revascularization						
Karlsson, et al,[12] 2019			NR	NR	NR	NR	NR	NR
LRP Study (Waksman, et al,[13] 2019)	NR	Noncluprit cardiac death, cardiac arrest, nonfatal MI, ACS, revascularization by CABG or PCI, and readmission to hospital for angina with more than 20% diameter stenosis progression	UA or MI requiring revascularization as defined in PROSPECT I[19]	2014 ACC/AHA Definition (TIA or Stroke)	2014 ACC/AHA and PROSPECT I[19] Definition	NR	All interventional cardiology methods for treatment of coronary artery disease and 2014 ACC/AHA Definition	2014 ACC/AHA Definition: Any death due to immediate cardiac cause (MI, low-output failure, fatal arrhythmia)
PROSPECT II (Erlinge, et al,[14] 2021)	NR	Cardiac death MI Unstable angina Progressive angina either requiring revascularization or with rapid lesion progression (defined in the appendix) arising from untreated, nonculprit lesions during follow-up	NR	Intracranial hemorrhage or nonhemorrhagic stroke that led to death	Third Universal Definition and SCAI criteria	Ischemic chest pain (or equivalent) at rest considered to be myocardial ischemia on final diagnosis and without elevation in cardiac biomarkers of necrosis	NR	The composite of sudden cardiac death, death due to acute myocardial infarction, death due to heart failure, death due to arrhythmia, or death not due to known vascular or non-CV causes

Abbreviations: NR, not reported.

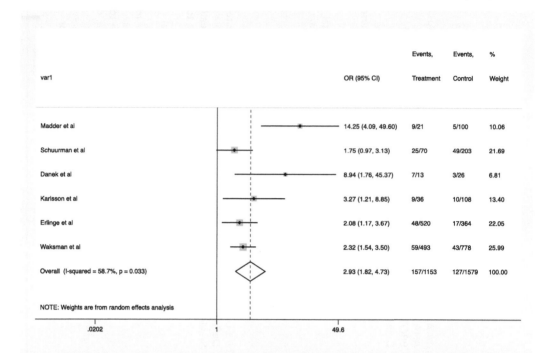

Fig. 2. Odds ratios and 95% confidence intervals for the occurrence of MACE/MACCE during follow-up after index presentation associated with all LCBI thresholds. The forest plot shows the results from the 6 included studies in the meta-analysis, listed by first author, along with the overall pooled summary estimate. The x-axis represents odds ratio values. The odds ratios and associated 95% confidence intervals are reported as a dot and line segment, respectively. The size of square data markers is proportional to the study weight in the meta-analysis. The summary measure point estimate and 95% confidence interval is represented as a diamond at the bottom of the plot. Number of events in the treatment group, defined as LCBI above threshold, and control group, defined as LCBI below threshold, used in the odds ratio calculations are provided on the right side of the table. All included study results suggest that LCBI values above the prespecified threshold was significantly associated with an increased odds of MACE/MACCE during follow-up. The thresholds used are as follows: $maxLCBI_{4mm} \geq 400$, $maxLCBI_{4mm} \geq 360$ (fourth quartile), $LCBI \geq 77$ (determined using receiver-operator characteristic analysis), $maxLCBI_{4mm} \geq 400$, $maxLCBI_{4mm} \geq 324.7$, and $maxLCBI_{4mm} > 400$ for Madder, Schuurman, Danek, Karlsson, Erlinge, and Waksman and colleagues, respectively.

Clinical Outcomes

The primary analysis and individual OR are shown in Fig. 2. The 6 included studies used different LCBI thresholds, ranging from LCBI of 77 or greater to LCBI of 400 or greater (specifically, $maxLCBI_{4mm}$). Overall, identification of vulnerable plaques with NIRS is associated with 2.93 times increased odds of MACE/MACCE (95% CI 1.82–4.73, $I^2 = 58.7\%$) in the pooled meta-analysis. Waksman and colleagues was weighted the most at 25.99%. Erlinge and colleagues was weighted the second highest at 22.05%.

The secondary outcome is shown in Fig. 3, which provides a forest plot depicting pooled results from studies using a max 4 mm LCBI threshold at or around 400. Studies included for the secondary endpoint were Madder and colleagues, Schuurman and colleagues, Karlsson and colleagues, Erlinge and colleagues, and Waksman and colleagues. Madder and colleagues, Karlsson

and colleagues, and Waksman and colleagues used 400 as the threshold $maxLCBI_{4mm}$. Schuurman and colleagues used $maxLCBI_{4mm}$ of 360 or greater and Erlinge and colleagues used $maxLCBI_{4mm}$ of 324.7 or greater as the primary analysis, both representing the upper quartile. The pooled odds ratio was 2.67 (95% CI 1.67–4.25, $I^2 = 58.4\%$). Waksman and colleagues and Erlinge and colleagues again were weighted the most at 28.79% and 23.85%, respectively.

Risk of Bias Assessment

All included studies were considered at high overall risk of bias.

DISCUSSION

Meta-Analysis Findings

This quantitative analysis showed that the detection of large lipid-rich plaque by NIRS is a powerful tool to predict major adverse CV

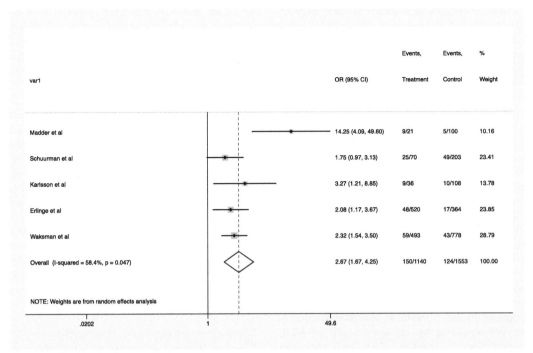

Fig. 3. Odds ratios and 95% confidence intervals for the occurrence of MACE/MACCE during follow-up after index presentation associated with maxLCBI$_{4mm}$ thresholds at or around 400. The forest plot shows the results from the 5 included studies in the meta-analysis, listed by first author, along with the overall pooled summary estimate. The x-axis represents odds ratio values. The odds ratios and associated 95% confidence intervals are reported as a dot and line segment, respectively. The size of square data markers is proportional to the study weight in the meta-analysis. The summary measure point estimate and 95% confidence interval is represented as a diamond at the bottom of the plot. Number of events in the treatment group, defined as maxLCBI$_{4mm}$ above threshold, and control group, defined as maxLCBI$_{4mm}$ below threshold, used in the odds ratio calculations are provided on the right side of the table. All included study results suggest that maxLCBI$_{4mm}$ values above the prespecified threshold was significantly associated with an increased odds of MACE/MACCE during follow-up. The thresholds used are as follows: maxLCBI$_{4mm}$ ≥ 400, maxLCBI$_{4mm}$ ≥ 360 (fourth quartile), maxLCBI$_{4mm}$ ≥ 400, maxLCBI$_{4mm}$ ≥ 324.7, and maxLCBI$_{4mm}$ > 400 for Madder, Schuurman, Karlsson, Erlinge, and Waksman and colleagues, respectively.

events in patients with coronary artery disease. The main contribution of this meta-analysis is the significantly improved precision of the pooled estimate odds ratio of 2.93 (95% CI 1.82–4.73) as seen in Fig. 2. The 95% CIs of the individual OR from each study were generally wider and more varied, with the narrowest interval of OR 1.54 to 3.50 in Waksman and colleagues and the widest interval of OR 1.76 to 45.37 in Danek and colleagues. The pooled estimate provides a narrow CI of OR 1.82 to 4.73. This more precise odds ratio with a narrow standard deviation of the relationship between lipid-rich plaques identified by NIRS and subsequent adverse events can be used in future studies to guide sample size calculations.

Furthermore, this meta-analysis confirms maxLCBI$_{4mm}$ of 400 or greater as an appropriate cutoff for identifying high-risk lipid rich plaques at the patient and individual plaque level. Similarly, it improves the precision of this cutoff in

predicting adverse events. The narrowest 95% CI of the 4 included studies was Waksman and colleagues from 1.54 to 3.50 while the widest interval was Madder and colleagues from 4.09 to 49.60. The pooled estimate from the meta-analysis provided an OR of 2.67 with a 95% CI of 1.67 to 4.25. This suggests that this is a reasonable binary cutoff to use in future studies.

Literature Review
Relationship between increasing lipid core burden index and adverse events
NIRS is a catheter-based intracoronary imaging technique that uses diffuse reflectance spectroscopy to measure the chemical signature of cholesterol within the coronary vessel wall. The specific molecular features of cholesterol lie within the near-infrared light wavelength region and can thus be distinguished from collagen to identify lipid-rich plaques from normal vessel or fibrotic and calcified plaques.[8] The technology

has been previously validated to detect lipid-rich plaque.[6,15] The studies included in this meta-analysis evaluate the effectiveness of NIRS as a tool to identify plaques and/or patients likely to experience future adverse events. It is hypothesized that detecting at-risk patients and prospectively treating vulnerable plaques could prevent future coronary events.

The predictive ability of NIRS has evolved from identification of vulnerable patients based on global lipid burden to identification of individual vulnerable plaques with the potential for secondary intervention. The earliest studies explored the prognostic value of identifying vulnerable patients based on findings of lipid-rich plaques without addressing the potential for plaque-level prognostic identification. However, these studies were relatively small and used different LCBI thresholds. Oemrawsingh and colleagues with a sample size of 203 patients was the first to identify the long-term prognostic value of NIRS as assessed in nonculprit vessels using an LCBI threshold of 43.0, representing the median.[8] The study reported a 1-year cumulative incidence of MACCE to be 16.7% in patients with an LCBI of 43 or greater versus 4.0% in those with an LCBI less than the threshold.

Schuurman and colleagues expanded on the findings of Oemrawsingh and colleagues, increasing the sample size to 275 by adding the IBIS-3-NIRS cohort to the original ATHEROREMO-NIRS cohort and increasing follow-up from 1-year to 4-year. The authors reported a statistically significant and independent continuous relationship between higher maxLCBI$_{4mm}$ values and a higher risk of MACE in a nontarget vessel using hazard ratios (HR). Each additional 100 units of maxLCBI$_{4mm}$ value was associated with a 19% increase in MACE (HR 1.19, 95% CI 1.07–1.32). This is similar to the findings from later studies such as Waksman and colleagues, which reported that there is an 18% increase in risk at the patient level for each 100-unit increase in maxLCBI$_{4mm}$ (HR 1.18, 95% CI 1.05–1.32) using a much larger sample size of 1271.

Waksman and colleagues further determined that NIRS can predict adverse outcomes at the individual plaque level by testing the association between maxLCBI$_{4mm}$ in a Ware segment, as defined in the study protocol, and occurrence of MACE within that same segment during the 24-month follow-up period. Waksman and colleagues showed each additional 100 units of maxLCBI$_{4mm}$ value at the plaque level was associated with a 45% increase in MACE (unadjusted

HR 1.45, 95% CI 1.3–1.60). Erlinge and colleagues similarly corroborated this relationship with a 4-year Kaplan-Meier estimated rate of events that showed an increase in nonculprit lesion-related MACE according to baseline maxLCBI$_{4mm}$ in increments of 100. Erlinge and colleagues showed a 3.7% increased site-specific risk of MACE during a 4-year period from index presentation in patients with maxLCBI$_{4mm}$ between 400 and 500, a 5.7% increase in patients with maxLCBI$_{4mm}$ between 500 and 600, and a 10.4% increased risk in patients with maxLCBI$_{4mm}$ more than 600. The ability to prospectively identify risk of particular lipid-rich plaques makes for more robust risk prediction. An example patient case emphasizing the role of NIRS in risk prediction, modified from Waksman and colleagues, is described in Fig. 1. Further research may explore opportunities for intervention and treatment at the plaque-level to prevent future coronary events.

Lipid core burden index as a marker for therapy efficacy and response to therapy

NIRS has also demonstrated an ability to assess plaque modification by new pharmacologic therapies. In the PACMAN-AMI randomized clinical trial recently published by Räber and colleagues,[16] NIRS-derived maxLCBI$_{4mm}$ was used to show the superiority of alirocumab in reducing lipid core burden when given in addition to high-intensity statin versus high-intensity statin therapy alone. Mean change in maxLCBI$_{4mm}$ was −79.42 with alirocumab plus rosuvastatin and −37.60 with rosuvastatin alone after 52 weeks of therapy in patients with acute myocardial infarction (difference, −41.24, $P = .006$).[16] Particularly when used in conjunction with other imaging modalities such as IVUS and optical coherence tomography, NIRS allowed for valuable plaque level characterization that can be used in future studies to help evaluate the efficacy of novel treatments that may minimize complications at follow-up. As options for secondary prevention become more robust and efficacious, NIRS will have increasing importance as a strategy for both identifying high-risk patients and quantifying their response to treatment.

Lipid core burden index best cutoff associated with cardiovascular events

There have been different values defining elevated LCBI. Oemrawsingh and colleagues defined values above that of the median (LCBI > 43 in their study) as an elevated LCBI, which is relatively similar to the definition used by Danek and colleagues (LCBI $\geq$ 77). Madder and colleagues, Karlsson and colleagues, and Waksman and colleagues define elevated LCBI as a maxLCBI$_{4mm}$ greater than 400 with Schuurman and colleagues choosing a similar value of any LCBI at or above the fourth quartile (maxLCBI$_{4mm}$ $\geq$ 360). Erlinge and colleagues used the upper quartile maxLCBI$_{4mm}$ of 324.7 as the prespecified definition of lipid-rich plaque. Erlinge and colleagues furthermore explored a different definition to define vulnerable plaques as any plaque with maxLCBI$_{4mm}$ in the highest quartile plus plaque burden greater than 70% or small luminal area (defined as $\leq$ 4 mm^2). We recommend to always use the LCBI value as a marker of continuum risk and maxLCBI$_{4mm}$ greater than 400 to categorize patients/plaques as a high risk.

Limitations
There are several limitations that must be acknowledged: First, reliability and validity of the WebPlotDigitizer program has been questioned in prior studies at an aggregate level.[17] However, results in a 2016 study indicated high levels of intercoder reliability and validity.[18] To minimize this limitation, we relied on reported numbers for odds ratio calculations whenever possible. Second, the primary outcomes for each study include a range of LCBI value thresholds to determine the OR. We conducted the secondary analysis including studies with maxLCBI$_{4mm}$ thresholds around 400 to optimize the comparison. Although the NIRS binary cutoff of 400 maxLCBI$_{4mm}$ was confirmed as a reasonable predictor for subsequent events at the patient and plaque level in Waksman and colleagues, a definitive optimal threshold has yet to be determined. Third, the longest length of follow-up was a median of 5.3 years, with the majority of the identified studies with less than 4 years of follow-up. Many of the studies might have missed important LCBI-related adverse events due to short follow-up. More research is needed to determine the incidence of adverse events over time. Finally, we recognize that there exists a moderate level of heterogeneity between studies, as delineated with the I^2 statistical (58.7%).

SUMMARY

NIRS-derived LCBI is an effective measurement for identifying vulnerable patients and plaques at risk of future MACE/MACCE. Patients with an elevated LCBI have 2.93 times higher odds of enduring a future adverse event. The precision of the pooled OR provides a more precise estimate that can be used in future studies. A

maxLCBI$_{4mm}$ of 400 or greater seems to be a useful threshold for classifying at-risk plaques.

CLINICS CARE POINTS

- NIRS can identify particular patients at risk for future MACE/MACCE and provide an opportunity for risk stratification.
- NIRS-derived maxLCBI$_{4mm}$ > 400 can locate high-risk lipid-rich plaques and predict potential areas of future complication.
- NIRS has demonstrated an ability to assess plaque modification by new pharmacologic therapies and quantify patient responsiveness to treatment.

DISCLOSURE

H M. Garcia-Garcia reports the following Institutional grant support: Biotronik, Boston Scientific, Medtronic, Abbott, Neovasc, Shockwave, Phillips and Corflow. R Waksman: Advisory Board: Amgen, Boston Scientific, Cardioset, Cardiovascular Systems Inc., Medtronic, Philips, Pi-Cardia Ltd.; Consultant: Amgen, Biotronik, Boston Scientific, Cardioset, Cardiovascular Systems Inc., Medtronic, Philips, Pi-Cardia Ltd.; Grant Support: AstraZeneca, United Kingdom; Biotronik, Germany; Boston Scientific, United States; Chiesi, Italy; Speakers Bureau: AstraZeneca, Chiesi, Italy; Investor: MedAlliance. P Shah and S Sum are employees of InfraRedx, A Nipro Company. Other authors do not have conflicts of interest.

ACKNOWLEDGMENTS

Thank you to all co-authors for their expertise and assistance throughout each aspect of this analysis and for their help in drafting and editing the manuscript.

REFERENCES

1. Virani SS, Alonso A, Benjamin EJ, et al. Heart disease and stroke statistics—2020 update: a report from the american heart association. Circulation 2020;141(9):e139–596.
2. Finn AV, Nakano M, Narula J, et al. Concept of Vulnerable/Unstable Plaque. Arterioscler Thromb Vasc Biol 2010;30(7):1282–92.
3. Muller JE, Abela GS, Nesto RW, et al. Triggers, acute risk factors and vulnerable plaques: the lexicon of a new frontier. J Am Coll Cardiol 1994; 23(3):809–13.

4. Virmani R, Kolodgie FD, Burke AP, et al. Lessons from sudden coronary death. Arterioscler Thromb Vasc Biol 2000;20(5):1262–75.

5. Wilkinson SE, Madder RD. Intracoronary near-infrared spectroscopy—role and clinical applications. Cardiovasc Diagn Ther 2020;10(5):1508–16.

6. Gardner CM, Tan H, Hull EL, et al. Detection of lipid core coronary plaques in autopsy specimens with a novel catheter-based near-infrared spectroscopy system. JACC: Cardiovasc Imaging 2008;1(5): 638–48.

7. Moher D, Liberati A, Tetzlaff J, et al. Preferred reporting items for systematic reviews and meta-analyses: The PRISMA statement. Int J Surg 2010; 8(5):336–41.

8. Oemrawsingh RM, Cheng JM, García-García HM, et al. Near-infrared spectroscopy predicts cardiovascular outcome in patients with coronary artery disease. J Am Coll Cardiol 2014;64(23):2510–8.

9. Madder RD, Husaini M, Davis AT, et al. Large lipid-rich coronary plaques detected by near-infrared spectroscopy at non-stented sites in the target artery identify patients likely to experience future major adverse cardiovascular events. Eur Heart J - Cardiovasc Imaging 2016;17(4):393–9.

10. Danek BA, Karatasakis A, Karacsonyi J, et al. Long-term follow-up after near-infrared spectroscopy coronary imaging: Insights from the lipid cORe plaque association with CLinical events (ORACLE-NIRS) registry. Cardiovasc Revascularization Med 2017;18(3):177–81.

11. Schuurman AS, Vroegindewey M, Kardys I, et al. Near-infrared spectroscopy-derived lipid core burden index predicts adverse cardiovascular outcome in patients with coronary artery disease during long-term follow-up. Eur Heart J 2018; 39(4):295–302.

12. Karlsson S, Anesäter E, Fransson K, et al. Intracoronary near-infrared spectroscopy and the risk of future cardiovascular events. Open Heart 2019; 6(1):e000917.

13. Waksman R, Mario CD, Torguson R, et al. Identification of patients and plaques vulnerable to future coronary events with near-infrared spectroscopy intravascular ultrasound imaging: a prospective, cohort study. Lancet 2019;394(10209): 1629–37.

14. Erlinge D, Maehara A, Ben-Yehuda O, et al. Identification of vulnerable plaques and patients by intracoronary near-infrared spectroscopy and ultrasound (PROSPECT II): a prospective natural history study. Lancet 2021;397(10278):985–95.

15. Waxman S, Dixon SR, L'Allier P, et al. In vivo validation of a catheter-based near-infrared spectroscopy system for detection of lipid core coronary plaques: initial results of the spectacl study. JACC: Cardiovasc Imaging 2009;2(7): 858–68.

16. Räber L, Ueki Y, Otsuka T, et al. Effect of alirocumab added to high-intensity statin therapy on coronary atherosclerosis in patients with acute myocardial infarction: the PACMAN-AMI randomized clinical trial. JAMA 2022. https://doi.org/10.1001/jama.2022.5218. Published online April 3.

17. Moeyaert M, Maggin D, Verkuilen J. Reliability, validity, and usability of data extraction programs for single-case research designs. Behav Modification 2016;40(6):874–900.

18. Drevon D, Fursa SR, Malcolm AL. Intercoder Reliability and validity of webplotdigitizer in extracting graphed data. Behav Modif 2017;41(2):323–39.

19. Stone GW, Maehara A, Lansky AJ, et al. A prospective natural-history study of coronary atherosclerosis. N Engl J Med 2011;364(3):226–35.

Near-Infrared Spectroscopy-Guided Percutaneous Coronary Intervention: Practical Applications and Available Evidence

Malav J. Parikh, MD, Ryan D. Madder, MD*

KEYWORDS

• Near-infrared spectroscopy • NIRS • Intracoronary imaging • Vulnerable plaque

---

KEY POINTS

- Intracoronary near-infrared spectroscopy (NIRS) has been extensively validated against the gold standard of histology to detect lipid-rich fibroatheroma.
- By detecting lipid-rich plaques in the coronary arteries, NIRS can identify vulnerable patients at increased risk of future patient-level cardiovascular events.
- NIRS can detect vulnerable plaques at increased risk of causing future site-specific coronary events.

BACKGROUND ON NEAR-INFRARED SPECTROSCOPY

Spectroscopy, the measurement of interaction of electromagnetic waves with matter, can identify the composition of a substance based on the varying amounts of absorption and scatter of emitted the electromagnetic waves.[1] Wavelengths just above the visible field of 800 to 2500 nm make up the near-infrared portion of the electromagnetic spectrum and are used by near-infrared spectroscopy (NIRS) to determine the composition of unknown substances.[1] The wavelengths used by NIRS are ideal for evaluating the composition of coronary plaques, particularly for detecting the presence of lipid-rich plaque (LRP) in a coronary artery.[1,2]

Invasive coronary angiography is the most commonly used modality to visualize disease in the coronary arteries. Although coronary angiography allows fluoroscopic visualization of the contrast-filled lumen, it does not provide characterization of plaque in the vessel walls. Unlike coronary angiography, intracoronary imaging modalities, including intravascular ultrasonography (IVUS) and optical coherence tomography (OCT), are capable of visualizing intracoronary plaque and can be used to assess plaque composition.[3] IVUS and OCT are both capable of detecting LRP, but detection of LRPs by these modalities is based on signal attenuation, thereby limiting their positive predictive value with regard to lipid-rich fibroatheroma detection.[4,5] In contrast, the detection of LRP by NIRS is based on the presence of the spectroscopic signature specific to intracoronary LRP.[6]

The NIRS system currently in clinical use, which combines NIRS and IVUS in a single

---

Frederik Meijer Heart & Vascular Institute, Spectrum Health, Grand Rapids, 100 Michigan Street Northeast, Grand Rapids, MI 49503, USA
* Corresponding author.
E-mail address: ryan.madder@spectrumhealth.org
Twitter: @RyanMadderMD (R.D.M.)

Intervent Cardiol Clin 12 (2023) 257–268
https://doi.org/10.1016/j.iccl.2022.10.007

catheter, is composed of a near-infrared laser, fiberoptic coronary catheter on a 3.2F monorail, automated pullback rotation device, and software to display the NIRS data.[7] This device is delivered over a standard coronary guidewire to a target location in a coronary artery. Upon initiating automated rotational pullback, 30,000 spectral measurements are made per 100 mm of artery scanned.[8] The NIRS data are then presented on a "chemogram," which is a 2-dimensional longitudinal map of the scanned vessel (Fig. 1). The chemogram uses a color scale transitioning from red to yellow as the probability of LRP increases, with pixels having a probability greater than 0.6 appearing yellow and those with lower probabilities appearing red.[1,7,8] A block chemogram is also created, which displays summary results for each 2-mm segment of the imaged artery (see Fig. 1). A numeric value is produced for each block, which corresponds to the 90th percentile of pixel values in the 2-mm segment. Each block is assigned 1 of 4 distinct colors to improve visual distinction based on the probability of LRP presence: red indicates probability less than 0.57, orange 0.57 to less than 0.84, tan 0.84 to less than or equal to 0.98, and yellow indicates probability greater than 0.98.[8] The lipid core burden index (LCBI), which provides a semiquantitative estimate of lipid burden, is calculated for any region of interest as the number of pixels having an LRP probability of 0.60 or greater divided by the number of valid pixels and then multiplying by 1000.[7] A commonly used metric to describe focal lipid core size is the maxLCBI$_{4mm}$, defined as the maximum LCBI in any 4-mm region of interest (Fig. 2).

Validation of Near-Infrared Spectroscopy Against Histopathology

Intracoronary NIRS has been validated for LRP detection in multiple studies against the gold standard of histopathology. Gardner and colleagues[6] originally validated NIRS in autopsied human hearts for the detection of a "lipid core plaque of interest," defined histologically in this study as a fibroatheroma with a lipid core greater than 60° in circumferential extent, greater than 200 μm thick, and with a fibrous cap having a mean thickness less than 450 μm. NIRS detected LRPs meeting these criteria with an area under the receiver operating curve of 0.80.[6] Subsequent studies have similarly validated NIRS findings against histology. Kang and colleagues[9] found that a yellow or tan block on the NIRS block chemogram identified

histologically proven fibroatheroma with a specificity of 94%. Puri and colleagues[10] found the combination of LCBI by NIRS and plaque burden by IVUS improved the diagnostic accuracy of fibroatheroma detection compared with either modality alone, thereby highlighting the benefits of multimodality intracoronary imaging. In a study evaluating the ability of NIRS to detect thin-capped fibroatheroma (TCFA), a maxLCBI$_{4mm}$ greater than or equal to 323 identified histologically proven TCFA with 80% sensitivity and 85% specificity.[11] NIRS imaging has also been studied in a diabetic and hypercholesterolemic porcine model in which NIRS-positive lesions were found by histology to be significantly more likely to have high-risk features including necrotic core, thin fibrous cap, and activated inflammatory cells.[12]

PRACTICAL APPLICATIONS
Use of Near-Infrared Spectroscopy Pre-PCI
Determining the mechanism of acute coronary syndromes
NIRS provides additional information over angiography regarding the characterization of culprit lesions and the mechanism underlying acute coronary syndrome (ACS). Postmortem studies of patients suffering fatal myocardial infarction (MI) demonstrated rupture of TCFA containing a large lipid core to be the mechanism triggering approximately two-thirds of cases.[13,14] Consistent with these findings, an early clinical study with NIRS demonstrated that culprit lesions in ACS more frequently harbored LRP compared with target lesions in stable coronary syndromes.[15] Early clinical studies with combined NIRS-IVUS in patients with STEMI, non-ST-elevation ACS, and sudden cardiac death showed that NIRS detected large LRP, characterized by a maxLCBI$_{4mm}$ greater than 400, in most culprit lesions.[16–18]

When used pre-percutaneous coronary intervention (PCI) to image culprit lesions in MI, NIRS-IVUS has recently been shown to accurately differentiate plaque rupture, plaque erosion, and calcified nodules as the underlying mechanism.[19] Using OCT as the reference standard, a threshold NIRS maxLCBI$_{4mm}$ of 426 at the culprit site accurately differentiated plaque rupture from erosion, with values greater than this threshold indicating plaque rupture. The algorithm developed and validated in this study is shown in Fig. 3.

Distinguishing plaque rupture from plaque erosion may be clinically significant, because PCI of lesions with plaque rupture associate with larger infarcts and more no-reflow and

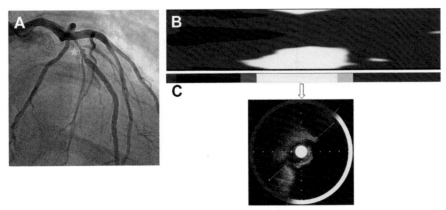

Fig. 1. NIRS chemogram and block chemogram. (*A*) Angiogram of a patient with ACS demonstrates a culprit lesion (*yellow star*) in the left anterior descending artery. (*B*) The corresponding NIRS chemogram (*top*) and block chemogram (*bottom*) are shown. The x-axis on the chemogram represents longitudinal position in the vessel. The y-axis represents circumferential position from 0° to 360°. Red regions represent low probability of LRP, and yellow regions represent high probability of LRP. Bright yellow blocks on the block chemogram represent regions having a greater than 98% probability of LRP presence. (*C*) Combined cross-sectional NIRS-IVUS image (*white arrow* shows location of cross-sectional image on the corresponding chemogram). The chemogram at this location is wrapped around the IVUS image, and the block chemogram at this location is in the central circle.

microvascular obstruction (MVO) compared with PCI of lesions with plaque erosion.[20] Patients with plaque rupture also have a higher risk of future cardiovascular events compared with those with plaque erosion.[21,22] The accurate identification of plaque erosion may eventually impact treatment decisions, as emerging data suggest a low event rate among some patients with MI caused by plaque erosion who are treated conservatively without stenting.[23–25]

Stent Length Selection

Ideally, the edges of an implanted stent should land in coronary segments free of significant atherosclerotic disease; however, angiography alone cannot accurately determine plaque-free landing zones. NIRS studies have shown that target lesion length is often underestimated by angiography, possibly leading to placement of a stent edge in an LRP resulting in a geographic miss.[26,27] In 2 small observational studies, NIRS

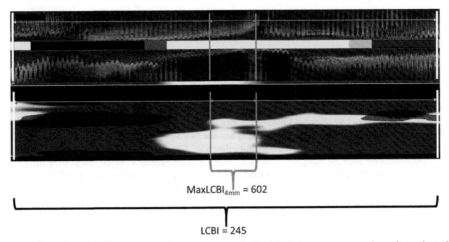

$MaxLCBI_{4mm} = 602$

$LCBI = 245$

Fig. 2. NIRS LCBI and $maxLCBI_{4mm}$. Any region of interest on the NIRS chemogram can be selected, and the software will automatically calculate the LCBI and $maxLCBI_{4mm}$ in the selected region. Here, a 37-mm segment of artery is selected as the region of interest (*white lines*). The LCBI is calculated as 245, which is the number of yellow pixels divided by the number of valid pixels in the region, multiplied by 1000. Within the region of interest, the $maxLCBI_{4mm}$ is automatically calculated by the software (*blue lines*), which is 602 in this case, thereby representing a relatively large LRP.

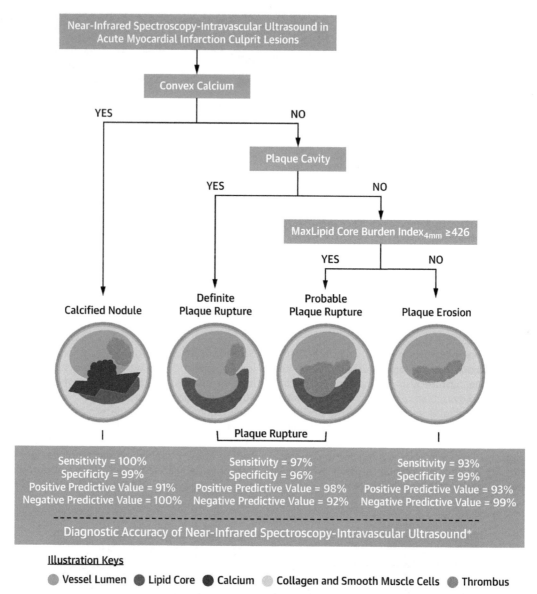

Fig. 3. NIRS-IVUS algorithm for determining cause of MI. The NIRS-IVUS classification algorithm classifies the culprit lesions of AMI in NIRS-IVUS-PR (including both definite and probable NIRS-IVUS-PR), NIRS-IVUS-PE, or NIRS-IVUS-CN. NIRS-IVUS-CN has convex calcium. Definite NIRS-IVUS-PR has plaque cavity. Probable NIRS-IVUS-PR has no plaque cavity but shows a high maxLCBI$_{4mm}$ of greater than or equal to 426. NIRS-IVUS-PE shows a low maxLCBI$_{4mm}$ of less than 426. *Diagnostic accuracy for NIRS-IVUS for identifying PR, PE, and CN was estimated in the validation cohort. AMI, acute myocardial infarction; CN, calcified nodule; PE, plaque erosion; PR, plaque rupture. (*Reproduced with* permission: Terada K, Kubo T, Kameyama T, et al. NIRS-IVUS for Differentiating Coronary Plaque Rupture, Erosion, and Calcified Nodule in Acute Myocardial Infarction. JACC Cardiovasc Imaging. 2021;14(7):1440-1450. Terada K. et al. J Am Coll Cardiol Img. 2021;14(7):1440-50.)

identified LRPs extending beyond the angiographic lesion margins in 16% to 52% of target lesions,[26,27] thereby highlighting the limitation of angiography alone in identifying disease-free landing zones for stent implantation.

Uncovered LRP in the stent margins may be clinically important, as Ino and colleagues[28]

found that LRP detected by OCT in the stent edge segments were associated with an increased risk of binary restenosis during follow-up. The risk of restenosis in this study depended on LRP size, such that larger LRPs were associated with significantly higher rates of restenosis. Alternatively, the NIRS maxLCBI$_{4mm}$ as measured post-PCI was not found in a recent observational study to be associated with the subsequent risk of target lesion failure (TLF).[29] However, it is important to note that in this single-center observational study, the residual lipid burden detected by NIRS within the stent margins was relatively small and large LRPs left uncovered in the stent margins were rare. Based on these limited available data, large LRPs left uncovered in the stent margins have been shown to associated with increased risk of events,[28] whereas the risk posed by smaller lipid cores may be minimal.[29] Further study of the clinical utility of NIRS imaging to inform decisions regarding stent length are warranted.

Predicting No Reflow and Periprocedural Myocardial Infarction

Performance of PCI on an LRP can result in distal embolization of plaque contents, MVO, no-reflow, and periprocedural MI, which are entities associated with adverse clinical outcomes.[30,31] A previous meta-analysis demonstrated an association between MVO and lower ejection fraction, larger ventricular volumes, and worse left ventricular remodeling.[32] Case reports in 2009 by Goldstein and colleagues[33] hypothesized that the detection of large LRPs by NIRS before PCI may predict the occurrence of no-reflow caused by distal embolization following PCI. Since then, LRPs detected by NIRS before PCI have been shown to be associated with periprocedural MI in several studies. Observational analysis of the CO-LOR registry discovered that large LRPs having a maxLCBI$_{4mm}$ greater than or equal to 500 were significantly associated with the occurrence of periprocedural MI. In this study, PCI of lesions having a maxLCBI$_{4mm}$ greater than or equal to 500 had a 50% rate of periprocedural MI and this threshold accurately differentiated lesions with and without periprocedural MI.[7] The CANARY trial subsequently found an increased likelihood of periprocedural MI when PCI was performed on LRPs having a maxLCBI$_{4mm}$ greater than or equal to 600.[34]

In a prospective NIRS-IVUS study of patients with STEMI, culprit lesion maxLCBI$_{4mm}$ was independently associated with the risk of MVO after primary PCI. The optimal threshold to differentiate lesions with and without MVO was a maxLCBI$_{4mm}$ greater than 600 (sensitivity 75%; specificity 69%).[35] In addition, the presence of MVO 1-week post-PCI as determined by cardiac MRI was associated with significantly lower left ventricular ejection fraction, greater infarct size, and increased ventricular volumes, mirroring previous studies.[32] These findings linking NIRS-detected LRP to no-reflow and periprocedural MI are in line with similar studies demonstrating the risk posed by LRP detected with other modalities such as OCT.[36,37]

Although NIRS findings before PCI have been shown to associate with the risk of adverse events, the prevention of periprocedural MI, distal embolization, MVO, and no-reflow when performing PCI on large LRP detected by NIRS has remained elusive. In the CANARY trial, the randomization of patients with large LRP to undergo PCI with or without a distal protection device did not show a difference in outcomes.[34] Additional studies are needed to delineate how periprocedural MI and no-reflow may be prevented when performing PCI on large LRP detected by NIRS.

Use of Near-Infrared Spectroscopy Post-PCI

Assessing residual lipid burden

A previous histologic study suggested an association between implantation of stent struts into a disrupted necrotic lipid core and subsequent stent thrombosis.[38] Further evidence that stent implantation into LRP might increase the risk of adverse events was demonstrated in a large OCT registry, in which irregular tissue protrusion post-PCI, an OCT finding believed to represent disrupted LRP, was associated with adverse events during follow-up.[39] Based on these prior histologic and OCT studies, it was hypothesized that retained LRP detected by NIRS in a stented segment may increase the risk of TLF during follow-up. In an observational study of patients undergoing PCI and having post-PCI NIRS-IVUS performed, the residual maxLCBI$_{4mm}$ detected by NIRS in the stented segment immediately after PCI was significantly associated with subsequent TLF, with an odds ratio of 1.6 for every 100-unit increase in the maxLCBI$_{4mm}$. It was determined that a residual maxLCBI$_{4mm}$ greater than 200 in the stented segment was the optimal threshold for identifying TLF over the 5-year study duration (sensitivity 81.2%; specificity 64.6%).[29] Confirmation of the association between residual lipid detected by NIRS immediately after stenting and the development of subsequent clinical events is warranted in additional studies.

Future Risk Assessment: Vulnerable Patient

Use of NIRS to image untreated coronary segments after PCI has been shown to identify vulnerable patients who are at a greater risk of patient-level cardiovascular events during follow-up. This fact was first demonstrated in an observational investigation, the ATHEROREMO-NIRS study, which showed that patients with an LCBI in a nonculprit vessel greater than or equal to the median value of 43 in the study population had a 4-fold higher risk of major adverse cardiovascular events (MACE) during follow-up.[40] Subsequently, a single-center observational study found that an NIRS-detected maxLCBI$_{4mm}$ greater than 400 at nonculprit sites within the culprit vessel was associated with a significantly increased risk of subsequent MACE. This study also suggested that patient-level risk may increase with increasing LRP size.[41] The ability of NIRS to identify vulnerable patients based on the maxLCBI$_{4mm}$ at nonculprit sites has since been demonstrated in several additional small observational studies.[42–44]

The first large multicenter study adequately powered to determine if NIRS could prospectively identify vulnerable patients was the Lipid Rich Plaque study, which followed 1271 patients with ACS or stable symptoms, who underwent NIRS-IVUS imaging of nonculprit coronary segments at baseline.[45] In this study, NIRS-IVUS was required to be performed in at least 2 major coronary arteries. During 24 months of follow-up, this study demonstrated the ability of NIRS to identify vulnerable patients, as every 100 unit increase in maxLCBI$_{4mm}$ was associated with an hazard ratio (HR) of 1.21 (95% confidence interval [CI], 1.09–1.35) for the development of nonculprit MACE ($P = .0004$) (Fig. 4). In addition, this study demonstrated a maxLCBI$_{4mm}$ threshold of 400 as a predictor of patient-level MACE risk with a HR of 2.18 (95% CI, 1.48–3.22; $P < .0001$).[45]

The PROSPECT II study also evaluated the ability of NIRS to identify patient-level cardiovascular risk.[46] In this study, patients with recent MI underwent 3-vessel NIRS-IVUS imaging after PCI was performed on all flow-limiting lesions. Patients were then followed for a median of 3.7 years. Among 898 patients, the presence of an untreated lesion having a maxLCBI$_{4mm}$ of 324.7 or greater, a threshold representing the upper quartile of maxLCBI$_{4mm}$ values in the study, was a marker of increased risk of patient-level MACE (odds ratio [OR], 2.08; 95% CI, 1.18–3.69). In a multivariable analysis that included both the NIRS and IVUS predictors of patient-level risk, a maxLCBI$_{4mm}$ of 324.7 or greater was independently predictive of patient-level MACE (adjusted OR, 3.80; 95% CI, 1.87–7.70) (Fig. 5).

Future Risk Assessment: Vulnerable Plaque
Using NIRS to identify vulnerable plaques at increased risk of causing future site-specific coronary event has been the subject of several recent studies. Previous cross-sectional studies of NIRS performed at the time of an ACS event demonstrated that NIRS frequently detects large LRP at culprit sites.[16–18,47] Furthermore, high maxLCBI$_{4mm}$ values had a high specificity for culprit sites in these studies. Based on these findings, it was postulated that the high NIRS maxLCBI$_{4mm}$ signal detected at the time of the ACS was likely present before the event and NIRS may therefore be capable of identifying vulnerable plaques before the ACS event occurs.[16,47]

The Lipid Rich Plaque Study, which as discussed earlier evaluated the ability of NIRS to identify vulnerable patients, also studied the ability of NIRS to identify vulnerable plaques.[45] In this prospective cohort study of 1271 ACS and stable patients followed for 2 years, nonculprit coronary segments at baseline having an increased lipid burden detected by NIRS were at increased risk of future site-specific coronary events. Every 100-unit increase in maxLCBI$_{4mm}$ had an HR of 1.45 (95% CI, 1.30–1.60) and an NIRS maxLCBI$_{4mm}$ greater than 400 at baseline had an HR of 4.22 (95% CI, 2.39–7.45) for future site-specific coronary events. Thus, the LRP study was the first to demonstrate that NIRS imaging is capable of detecting vulnerable plaques at increased risk of triggering future site-specific coronary events and is currently the only instrument with a US Food and Drug Administration label claim for vulnerable plaque detection.

More recently, the PROSPECT II study also demonstrated the ability of NIRS imaging to prospectively identify vulnerable plaques in a cohort of patients with recent MI. This prospective multicenter study recruited patients with recent MI and performed 3-vessel NIRS-IVUS imaging following treatment of all flow-limiting coronary lesions. During a median follow-up of 3.7 years, lesions having a maxLCBI$_{4mm}$ of 324.7 or greater at baseline, representing the upper quartile of maxLCBI$_{4mm}$ values, had a significantly increased risk of future site-specific coronary events (OR, 7.83; 95% CI, 4.12–14.89). Similar to the PROSPECT I study,[48] a plaque burden by IVUS of 70% or greater in PROSPECT II was also identified as an independent predictor of site-specific events. Lesions at baseline having both an NIRS maxLCBI$_{4mm}$ of 324.7 or greater and a plaque burden by IVUS of 70% or greater had a lesion-specific event rate during follow-up of 7%.[46]

The ability for NIRS imaging to identify vulnerable plaques in 2 large prospective multicenter studies raises questions regarding how this information might change clinical management of

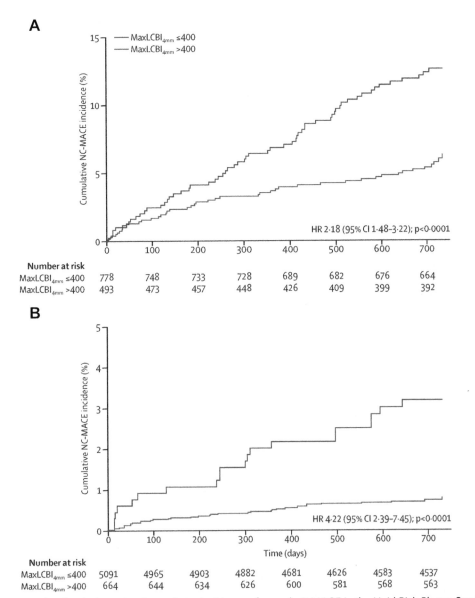

Fig. 4. Patient-level and plaque-level cumulative incidence of nonculprit MACE in the Lipid Rich Plaque Study. (*A*) Patient-level cumulative incidence of nonculprit MACE for coronary segments with and without a maxLCBI$_{4mm}$ of greater than 400. (*B*) Plaque-level cumulative incidence of nonculprit MACE for coronary segments with and without a maxLCBI$_{4mm}$ of greater than 400. NC-MACE = nonculprit major adverse cardiovascular events. (Reprinted with permission from Elsevier. The Lancet, Nov 2019, 394 (10209), 1629-1637.)

these lesions and the patients that harbor them. As both stent technology and pharmacotherapy advance, identifying vulnerable plaques may lead to a paradigm shift of more personalized coronary artery disease therapies for secondary prevention. The PROSPECT II ABSORB study recently evaluated the potential benefits of preemptive stenting of nonobstructive high-risk plaques detected by NIRS-IVUS.[49] In this pilot randomized controlled trial, a subset of 182

patients with recent MI enrolled in PROSEPCT II and found to have at least 1 plaque having a plaque burden of 65% or greater were randomized to undergo preemptive stenting with a bioresorbable vascular scaffold plus medical therapy or medical therapy alone. Repeat angiography and NIRS-IVUS imaging were performed on all patients at 25 months. The primary effectiveness endpoint was minimum lumen area (MLA), and the primary safety

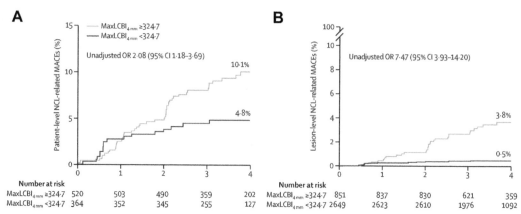

Fig. 5. Kaplan-Meier time-to-first-event curves for NCL-related MACEs according to presence of high-risk plaques in the PROSPECT II study. (A) Patient-level NCL-related MACE in patients with 1 or more baseline NCLs with high lipid content defined as maxLCBI greater than or equal to 324.7 compared with patients without any NCLs with high lipid content. (B) Lesion-level outcomes attributable to individual NCLs with high lipid content defined as maxLCBI greater than or equal to 324.7 compared with lesions without high lipid content. NCL, nonculprit lesions. (Reprinted with permission from Elsevier. The Lancet, Mar 2021, 397 (10278), 985-995.)

endpoint was TLF. Randomized lesions in this study were angiographically mild, having a median diameter stenosis of only 41.6% and were characterized by a large plaque burden (median 73.7%) and by a median $maxLCBI_{4mm}$ of 334. The MLA during follow-up was significantly greater among lesions undergoing preemptive PCI (MLA 6.9 ± 2.6 mm^2 vs 3.0 ± 1.0 mm^2, $P < .0001$). Rates of TLF were not significantly different among groups during follow-up (4.3% vs 4.5%, $P = .96$). Although not powered for hypothesis testing of clinical endpoints, the preemptive stenting group trended toward a reduced secondary outcome measure of cardiac death, target vessel-related MI, or target lesion revascularization (4.7% vs 10.7%; $P = .12$).[49] The results of this study demonstrate, for the first time, that PCI of angiographically mild lesions with high-risk features identified on NIRS-IVUS imaging is safe and results in larger MLA during follow-up. These findings will likely be used to inform future clinical outcomes studies of preemptive intervention of lesions with high-risk features. Notably, additional studies of preemptive stenting of vulnerable plaques are currently underway.[50]

Emerging Applications of Near-Infrared Spectroscopy Imaging
Assessing neoatherosclerosis in previously implanted stents
Neoatherosclerosis, the development of LRP within the neointima of previously placed coronary stents, has become a recognized cause of late and very late stent failure in recent years.[51] Originally described in postmortem studies, neoatherosclerosis can now be detected in vivo using various intracoronary imaging modalities.[52–59] Detection of neoatherosclerosis with NIRS was studied in an observational registry,[57] which compared NIRS-IVUS findings in preexisting stents with a control group of newly implanted stents. Among these 2 groups, NIRS findings did not differ, concluding that NIRS alone, because of its inability to determine the depth of a lipid signal, was unable to differentiate LRP under a stent from neoatherosclerosis. However, the combination of NIRS with IVUS may make detection of neoatherosclerosis possible.[52,57]

Assessing Coronary Allograft Vasculopathy
Coronary allograft vasculopathy (CAV) is a fibroproliferative process leading to luminal obstruction in the coronary arteries of transplanted hearts and is the leading cause of mortality after the first year of receiving a cardiac transplant.[60,61] There has been recent interest to use NIRS imaging to improve the detection and characterization of CAV. A study evaluating NIRS-IVUS characteristics of CAV compared with native atherosclerosis found that in segments with plaque burden less than 40% by IVUS, the NIRS $maxLCBI_{4mm}$ was greater in transplanted when compared with native arteries.[61] Further investigation is needed to understand the clinical implications of NIRS imaging in the detection of CAV.

Near-Infrared Spectroscopy as a Tool to Measure Effects of Novel Therapies

NIRS imaging may be useful to evaluate the effects of novel pharmacotherapeutics on LRP in the coronary arteries. Recently, Räber and colleagues[62] used NIRS for a secondary endpoint in a randomized control trial investigating the efficacy of alirocumab added to high-intensity statin and found a significant reduction in maxLCBI$_{4mm}$ in the alirocumab group at 1 year after AMI in noninfarct arteries. As shown in this study, using NIRS imaging may be useful to provide insight into the impact of novel therapies on vulnerable plaque and vulnerable patients. Future studies will likely use NIRS in this regard.

SUMMARY

NIRS has been extensively validated against the gold standard of histopathology to identify LRP and now has several practical applications when used both pre-PCI and post-PCI. When used pre-PCI, NIRS has clinical utility in determining the mechanism underlying ACS, can be used to guide stent length selection, and can identify the risk of periprocedural MI. When used post-PCI, NIRS can identify both vulnerable patients and vulnerable plaques. NIRS also has an emerging role in assessing the effects of novel therapies on lipid burden in the coronary arteries.

CLINICS CARE POINTS

- Large lipid-rich plaques detected by NIRS are associated with a greater risk of periprocedural myocardial infarction and no-reflow during PCI.
- Large lipid-rich plaques detected by NIRS at non-culprit sites are associated with a greater future risk of site-specific and patient-level adverse events.

DISCLOSURE

Dr R.D. Madder serves on the advisory board of SpectraWave and has received research support and serves as a consultant for Infraredx. Dr M.J. Parikh has nothing to disclose.

REFERENCES

1. Su JL, Grainger SJ, Greiner CA, et al. Detection and structural characterization of lipid-core plaques with intravascular NIRS-IVUS imaging. Interv Cardiol 2015;7(6):519–35.
2. Danek BA, Karatasakis A, Madder RD, et al. Experience with the multimodality near-infrared spectroscopy/intravascular ultrasound coronary imaging system: principles, clinical experience, and ongoing studies. Curr Cardiovasc Imaging Rep 2016;9(2):1–13.
3. Mintz GS. Clinical utility of intravascular imaging and physiology in coronary artery disease. J Am Coll Cardiol 2014;64(2):207–22.
4. Di Vito L, Imola F, Gatto L, et al. Limitations of OCT in identifying and quantifying lipid components: an in vivo comparison study with IVUS-NIRS. EuroIntervention: J EuroPCR collaboration Working Group Interv Cardiol Eur Soc Cardiol 2017;13(3): 303–11.
5. Fujii K, Hao H, Shibuya M, et al. Accuracy of OCT, grayscale IVUS, and their combination for the diagnosis of coronary TCFA: an ex vivo validation study. JACC Cardiovasc Imaging 2015;8(4):451–60.
6. Gardner CM, Tan H, Hull EL, et al. Detection of lipid core coronary plaques in autopsy specimens with a novel catheter-based near-infrared spectroscopy system. JACC Cardiovasc Imaging 2008;1(5): 638–48.
7. Goldstein JA, Maini B, Dixon SR, et al. Detection of lipid-core plaques by intracoronary near-infrared spectroscopy identifies high risk of periprocedural myocardial infarction. Circ Cardiovasc Interv 2011; 4(5):429–37.
8. Wilkinson SE, Madder RD. Intracoronary near-infrared spectroscopy-role and clinical applications. Cardiovasc Diagn Ther 2020;10(5):1508–16.
9. Kang SJ, Mintz GS, Pu J, et al. Combined IVUS and NIRS detection of fibroatheromas: histopathological validation in human coronary arteries. JACC Cardiovasc Imaging 2015;8(2):184–94.
10. Puri R, Madder RD, Madden SP, et al. Near-Infrared Spectroscopy Enhances Intravascular Ultrasound Assessment of Vulnerable Coronary Plaque: A Combined Pathological and In Vivo Study. Arterioscler Thromb Vasc Biol 2015;35(11): 2423–31.
11. Inaba S, Mintz GS, Burke AP, et al. Intravascular Ultrasound and Near-Infrared Spectroscopic Characterization of Thin-Cap Fibroatheroma. Am J Cardiol 2017;119(3):372–8.
12. Patel D, Hamamdzic D, Llano R, et al. Subsequent development of fibroatheromas with inflamed fibrous caps can be predicted by intracoronary near infrared spectroscopy. Arterioscler Thromb Vasc Biol 2013;33(2):347–53.
13. Burke AP, Farb A, Malcom GT, et al. Coronary risk factors and plaque morphology in men with coronary disease who died suddenly. New Engl J Med 1997;336(18):1276–82.

14. Virmani R, Kolodgie FD, Burke AP, et al. Lessons from sudden coronary death: a comprehensive morphological classification scheme for atherosclerotic lesions. Arteriosclerosis, Thromb Vasc Biol 2000;20(5):1262–75.

15. Madder RD, Smith JL, Dixon SR, et al. Composition of target lesions by near-infrared spectroscopy in patients with acute coronary syndrome versus stable angina. Circ Cardiovasc Interventions 2012; 5(1):55–61.

16. Madder RD, Goldstein JA, Madden SP, et al. Detection by near-infrared spectroscopy of large lipid core plaques at culprit sites in patients with acute ST-segment elevation myocardial infarction. JACC: Cardiovasc Interventions 2013;6(8): 838–46.

17. Madder RD, Wohns DH, Muller JE. Detection by intracoronary near-infrared spectroscopy of lipid core plaque at culprit sites in survivors of cardiac arrest. Card Imaging 2014;26(2):78–9.

18. Madder RD, Husaini M, Davis AT, et al. Detection by near-infrared spectroscopy of large lipid cores at culprit sites in patients with non-st-segment elevation myocardial infarction and unstable angina. Catheterization Cardiovasc Interventions 2015;86(6):1014–21.

19. Terada K, Kubo T, Kameyama T, et al. NIRS-IVUS for Differentiating Coronary Plaque Rupture, Erosion, and Calcified Nodule in Acute Myocardial Infarction. JACC Cardiovasc Imaging 2021;14(7): 1440–50.

20. Satogami K, Ino Y, Kubo T, et al. Impact of Plaque Rupture Detected by Optical Coherence Tomography on Transmural Extent of Infarction After Successful Stenting in ST-Segment Elevation Acute Myocardial Infarction. JACC Cardiovasc Interv 2017;10(10):1025–33.

21. Hayashi T, Kiyoshima T, Matsuura M, et al. Plaque erosion in the culprit lesion is prone to develop a smaller myocardial infarction size compared with plaque rupture. Am Heart J 2005;149(2):284–90.

22. Kusama I, Hibi K, Kosuge M, et al. Impact of plaque rupture on infarct size in ST-segment elevation anterior acute myocardial infarction. J Am Coll Cardiol 2007;50(13):1230–7.

23. Hu S, Zhu Y, Zhang Y, et al. Management and outcome of patients with acute coronary syndrome caused by plaque rupture versus plaque erosion: an intravascular optical coherence tomography study. J Am Heart Assoc 2017;6(3):e004730.

24. Jia H, Dai J, Hou J, et al. Effective anti-thrombotic therapy without stenting: intravascular optical coherence tomography-based management in plaque erosion (the EROSION study). Eur Heart J 2017;38(11):792–800.

25. Prati F, Uemura S, Souteyrand G, et al. OCT-based diagnosis and management of STEMI associated with intact fibrous cap. JACC: Cardiovasc Imaging 2013;6(3):283–7.

26. Hanson ID, Goldstein JA, Dixon SR, et al. Comparison of coronary artery lesion length by NIRS-IVUS versus angiography alone. Coron Artery Dis 2015; 26(6):484–9.

27. Dixon SR, Grines CL, Munir A, et al. Analysis of target lesion length before coronary artery stenting using angiography and near-infrared spectroscopy versus angiography alone. Am J Cardiol 2012; 109(1):60–6.

28. Ino Y, Kubo T, Matsuo Y, et al. Optical Coherence Tomography Predictors for Edge Restenosis After Everolimus-Eluting Stent Implantation. Circ Cardiovasc Interv 2016;9(10):e004231.

29. Madder RD, Kubo T, Ino Y, et al. Target Lesion Lipid Content Detected by Near-Infrared Spectroscopy After Stenting and the Risk of Subsequent Target Lesion Failure. Arterioscler Thromb Vasc Biol 2021;41(7):2181–9.

30. Morishima I, Sone T, Okumura K, et al. Angiographic no-reflow phenomenon as a predictor of adverse long-term outcome in patients treated with percutaneous transluminal coronary angioplasty for first acute myocardial infarction. J Am Coll Cardiol 2000;36(4):1202–9.

31. Ndrepepa G, Tiroch K, Fusaro M, et al. 5-year prognostic value of no-reflow phenomenon after percutaneous coronary intervention in patients with acute myocardial infarction. J Am Coll Cardiol 2010;55(21):2383–9.

32. Hamirani YS, Wong A, Kramer CM, et al. Effect of microvascular obstruction and intramyocardial hemorrhage by CMR on LV remodeling and outcomes after myocardial infarction: a systematic review and meta-analysis. JACC Cardiovasc Imaging 2014;7(9):940–52.

33. Goldstein JA, Grines C, Fischell T, et al. Coronary embolization following balloon dilation of lipid-core plaques. JACC Cardiovasc Imaging 2009; 2(12):1420–4.

34. Stone GW, Maehara A, Muller JE, et al. Plaque Characterization to Inform the Prediction and Prevention of Periprocedural Myocardial Infarction During Percutaneous Coronary Intervention: The CANARY Trial (Coronary Assessment by Near-infrared of Atherosclerotic Rupture-prone Yellow). JACC Cardiovasc Interv 2015;8(7):927–36.

35. Terada K, Kubo T, Madder RD, et al. Near-infrared spectroscopy to predict microvascular obstruction after primary percutaneous coronary intervention. EuroIntervention 2021;17(12):e999–1006.

36. Lee T, Yonetsu T, Koura K, et al. Impact of coronary plaque morphology assessed by optical coherence tomography on cardiac troponin elevation in patients with elective stent implantation. Circ Cardiovasc Interventions 2011;4(4):378–86.

37. Porto I, Di Vito L, Burzotta F, et al. Predictors of periprocedural (type IVa) myocardial infarction, as assessed by frequency-domain optical coherence tomography. Circ Cardiovasc Interventions 2012; 5(1):89–96.

38. Nakano M, Yahagi K, Otsuka F, et al. Causes of early stent thrombosis in patients presenting with acute coronary syndrome: an ex vivo human autopsy study. J Am Coll Cardiol 2014;63(23): 2510–20.

39. Soeda T, Uemura S, Park S-J, et al. Incidence and clinical significance of poststent optical coherence tomography findings: one-year follow-up study from a multicenter registry. Circulation 2015; 132(11):1020–9.

40. Oemrawsingh RM, Cheng JM, García-García HM, et al. Near-infrared spectroscopy predicts cardiovascular outcome in patients with coronary artery disease. J Am Coll Cardiol 2014;64(23):2510–8.

41. Madder RD, Husaini M, Davis AT, et al. Large lipid-rich coronary plaques detected by near-infrared spectroscopy at non-stented sites in the target artery identify patients likely to experience future major adverse cardiovascular events. Eur Heart J Cardiovasc Imaging 2016;17(4):393–9.

42. Schuurman A-S, Vroegindewey M, Kardys I, et al. Near-infrared spectroscopy-derived lipid core burden index predicts adverse cardiovascular outcome in patients with coronary artery disease during long-term follow-up. Eur Heart J 2018; 39(4):295–302.

43. Danek BA, Karatasakis A, Karacsonyi J, et al. Long-term follow-up after near-infrared spectroscopy coronary imaging: Insights from the lipid cORe plaque association with CLinical events (ORACLE-NIRS) registry. Cardiovasc Revascularization Med 2017;18(3):177–81.

44. Karlsson S, Anesäter E, Fransson K, et al. Intracoronary near-infrared spectroscopy and the risk of future cardiovascular events. Open Heart 2019; 6(1):e000917.

45. Waksman R, Di Mario C, Torguson R, et al. Identification of patients and plaques vulnerable to future coronary events with near-infrared spectroscopy intravascular ultrasound imaging: a prospective, cohort study. Lancet 2019;394(10209):1629–37.

46. Erlinge D, Maehara A, Ben-Yehuda O, et al. Identification of vulnerable plaques and patients by intracoronary near-infrared spectroscopy and ultrasound (PROSPECT II): a prospective natural history study. Lancet 2021;397(10278):985–95.

47. Madder RD, Puri R, Muller JE, et al. Confirmation of the intracoronary near-infrared spectroscopy threshold of lipid-rich plaques that underlie ST-segment–elevation myocardial infarction. Arteriosclerosis, Thromb Vasc Biol 2016;36(5):1010–5.

48. Stone GW, Maehara A, Lansky AJ, et al. A prospective natural-history study of coronary atherosclerosis. N Engl J Med 2011;364(3):226–35.

49. Stone GW, Maehara A, Ali ZA, et al. Percutaneous Coronary Intervention for Vulnerable Coronary Atherosclerotic Plaque. J Am Coll Cardiol 2020; 76(20):2289–301.

50. The Preventive Coronary Intervention on Stenosis With Functionally Insignificant Vulnerable Plaque. https://ClinicalTrials.gov/show/NCT02316886. [Accessed 26 November 2022].

51. Otsuka F, Byrne RA, Yahagi K, et al. Neoatherosclerosis: overview of histopathologic findings and implications for intravascular imaging assessment. Eur Heart J 2015;36(32):2147–59.

52. Ali ZA, Roleder T, Narula J, et al. Increased thin-cap neoatheroma and periprocedural myocardial infarction in drug-eluting stent restenosis: multimodality intravascular imaging of drug-eluting and bare-metal stents. Circ Cardiovasc Interventions 2013;6(5):507–17.

53. Habara M, Terashima M, Suzuki T. Detection of atherosclerotic progression with rupture of degenerated in-stent intima five years after bare-metal stent implantation using optical coherence tomography. J invasive Cardiol 2009;21(10):552–3.

54. Kang S-J, Mintz GS, Akasaka T, et al. Optical coherence tomographic analysis of in-stent neoatherosclerosis after drug–eluting stent implantation. Circulation 2011;123(25):2954–63.

55. Kang S-J, Mintz GS, Park D-W, et al. Tissue characterization of in-stent neointima using intravascular ultrasound radiofrequency data analysis. Am J Cardiol 2010;106(11):1561–5.

56. Lee CW, Kang S-J, Park D-W, et al. Intravascular ultrasound findings in patients with very late stent thrombosis after either drug-eluting or bare-metal stent implantation. J Am Coll Cardiol 2010;55(18):1936–42.

57. Madder RD, Khan M, Husaini M, et al. Combined Near-Infrared Spectroscopy and Intravascular Ultrasound Imaging of Pre-Existing Coronary Artery Stents: Can Near-Infrared Spectroscopy Reliably Detect Neoatherosclerosis? Circ Cardiovasc Imaging 2016;9(1):e003576.

58. Takano M, Yamamoto M, Inami S, et al. Appearance of lipid-laden intima and neovascularization after implantation of bare-metal stents: extended late-phase observation by intracoronary optical coherence tomography. J Am Coll Cardiol 2009; 55(1):26–32.

59. Yokoyama S, Takano M, Yamamoto M, et al. Extended follow-up by serial angioscopic observation for bare-metal stents in native coronary arteries: from healing response to atherosclerotic transformation of neointima. Circ Cardiovasc Interventions 2009;2(3):205–12.

60. Pollack A, Nazif T, Mancini D, et al. Detection and imaging of cardiac allograft vasculopathy. JACC Cardiovasc Imaging 2013;6(5):613–23.

61. Zheng B, Maehara A, Mintz GS, et al. In vivo comparison between cardiac allograft vasculopathy and native atherosclerosis using near-infrared spectroscopy and intravascular ultrasound. Eur Heart J Cardiovasc Imaging 2015;16(9):985–91.

62. Räber L, Ueki Y, Otsuka T, et al. Effect of Alirocumab Added to High-Intensity Statin Therapy on Coronary Atherosclerosis in Patients With Acute Myocardial Infarction: The PACMAN-AMI Randomized Clinical Trial. JAMA 2022;327(18):1771–81.

Invasive Intracoronary Imaging of Cardiac Allograft Vasculopathy: Established Modalities and Emerging Technologies

Negeen Shahandeh, MD[a], Rushi V. Parikh, MD[b],*

KEYWORDS

- Cardiac allograft vasculopathy • Heart transplantation • Intravascular imaging
- Intravascular ultrasound • Optical coherence tomography • Near-infrared spectroscopy

---

KEY POINTS

- Cardiac allograft vasculopathy (CAV) is a major cause of adverse clinical outcomes among heart transplant recipients
- Invasive intracoronary imaging is a vital adjunct to coronary angiography for the early diagnosis of CAV
- Multiple studies have demonstrated the prognostic value of intravascular ultrasound metrics of CAV among heart transplant patients
- Emerging invasive intracoronary imaging modalities currently lack outcome data but have the potential to further elucidate CAV pathophysiology and identify novel therapeutic targets

---

INTRODUCTION

Christiaan Barnard performed the first human-to-human heart transplant in South Africa in 1967.[1] More than 50 years later, many advances in heart transplantation have led to increased survival and quality of life for the nearly 6000 heart transplant recipients annually worldwide.[2] Cardiac allograft vasculopathy (CAV), a complex fibroproliferative disease of the allograft coronary circulation, remains a leading cause of long-term mortality, accounting for roughly 10% of deaths annually after the first year post-transplant.[2,3] In particular, those who develop accelerate disease within the first year after transplant have markedly worse rates of death or graft failure at 5 years.[4,5]

Despite measures to prevent and/or attenuate CAV such as early initiation of statins, infectious prophylaxis, and treatment of acute rejection, CAV continues to affect approximately 30% of allografts by 5 years after transplant and nearly 50% of allografts by 10 years after transplant in the current era (Fig. 1).[2,6,7] Moreover, recent international registry data demonstrate only mild improvement in 5-year survival from CAV (Fig. 2).[2,7] These sobering data may be partly explained by the fact that denervated heart transplant recipients often do not develop angina and therefore may present with late-stage manifestations of CAV including silent myocardial infarction, graft failure, or sudden cardiac death. For this reason, regular screening

---

[a] Division of Cardiology, University of California, 100 Medical Plaza, Suite 630 East, Los Angeles, CA 90095, USA;
[b] Division of Cardiology, University of California, Los Angeles, 100 Medical Plaza, Suite 630 West, Los Angeles, CA 90095; USA
* Corresponding author.
E-mail address: rparikh@mednet.ucla.edu
Twitter: @rushiparikh11 (R.V.P.)

Intervent Cardiol Clin 12 (2023) 269–280
https://doi.org/10.1016/j.iccl.2022.12.005
2211-7458/23/© 2022 Elsevier Inc. All rights reserved.

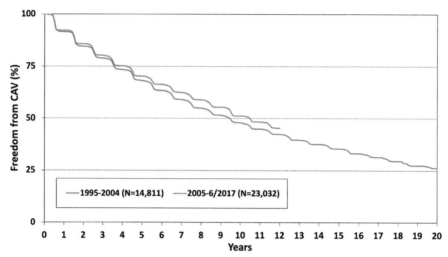

Fig. 1. Freedom from CAV. Comparison of CAV incidence by era of heart transplantation shows only mild increase in the rate of freedom from CAV at annual follow-up. (Reproduced and adapted with permission from the 2019 ISHLT Registry Report (ISHLT 2019 REGISTRY REPORT JHLT. 2019 Oct; 38(10): 1015-1066).

for CAV with coronary angiography is the current standard of care, and more sensitive intravascular imaging platforms that can detect CAV at earlier stages than angiography are increasingly being used in conjunction and studied with the goal of instituting effective treatment to prevent and/or slow disease progression sooner after transplant.[8] Intracoronary imaging technologies provide more detailed characterization of CAV lesions, and these novel insights into the pathophysiology of CAV have the potential to identify new

therapeutic targets and assess response to treatment. The present review will highlight the current and emerging invasive imaging modalities available for use in diagnosing and characterizing CAV and the data supporting each platform.

PATHOPHYSIOLOGY OF CARDIAC ALLOGRAFT VASCULOPATHY

CAV is a unique form of fibroproliferative coronary artery disease that affects the epicardial

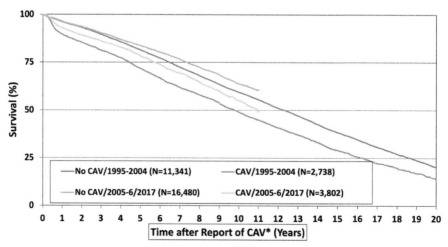

Fig. 2. Survival after diagnosis of CAV. Survival rate after a diagnosis of CAV within the first 3 years after transplantation, stratified by era. * Patient survival for those without CAV within 3 years after transplant was conditioned on survival to median time of CAV development (518 days). Median time to CAV development is based on patients who developed CAV within 3 years of transplant. (Reproduced and adapted with permission from the 2019 ISHLT Registry Report (ISHLT 2019 REGISTRY REPORT JHLT. 2019 Oct; 38(10): 1015-1066).

and microvascular circuits of transplanted hearts. Specifically, it is distinguished by diffuse intimal hyperplasia and negative remodeling (characterized by heightened medial tone and adventitial fibrosis), leading to accelerated luminal narrowing (Fig. 3). Over time, luminal compromise and decreased coronary blood flow eventually manifest as graft failure. Histologic findings include smooth muscle proliferation, lipid deposition, and accumulation of inflammatory cells.[9] These processes are now understood to be mediated by both immunologic and nonimmunologic factors.[6,8]

Alloantigen and foreign human leukocyte antigen (HLA) presentation by host immune cells results in T-cell activation and the release of proinflammatory cytokines. The downstream effects of this inflammatory cascade include upregulation of adhesion molecules by endothelial cells and recruitment of macrophages, which further perpetuate inflammation and fibrosis, ultimately leading to smooth muscle proliferation in the intima.[10] Immune-mediated risk factors include higher number of HLA mismatches, HLA-DR mismatch, presence of donor-specific antibodies, and history of antibody-mediated rejection. In addition to immune-mediated risk factors, traditional cardiovascular risk factors also promote vascular endothelial inflammation and contribute to the development of CAV. Cytomegalovirus (CMV) infection has also been associated with the development of CAV. Although the mechanism by which CMV infection increases the risk for CAV is not fully understood, proposed hypotheses include molecular mimicry and direct endothelial damage mediated by dysfunction of the nitric oxide synthase pathway.[11] Furthermore, any process that results in tissue damage such as ischemia-reperfusion injury or donor brain death can result in an inflammatory milieu that promotes CAV.[10]

LIMITATIONS OF NONINVASIVE IMAGING

Noninvasive imaging modalities for CAV surveillance are attractive due to their ability to limit procedural risk. Several noninvasive tests have been studied in this arena, including dobutamine stress echocardiography (DSE), single-photon emission computed tomography (SPECT), positron-emission tomography (PET), coronary computed tomography angiography, and cardiac magnetic resonance imaging.[12–15] Although many of these modalities demonstrate a high specificity for diagnosing CAV, they are unable to evaluate the vessel wall and hence are significantly less sensitive for detecting early

CAV than invasive imaging modalities. For example, one study combining resting echocardiography with dipyridamole SPECT demonstrated a specificity of 83% for detecting CAV while only achieving a sensitivity of 60%.[12] Similarly, although the historically reported sensitivity of DSE is 65%, a contemporary study of 497 transplant recipients who underwent both coronary angiography and DSE revealed only a 7% sensitivity for the detection of CAV.[16] Cardiac PET, which allows for quantification of myocardial blood flow and flow reserve, has shown promise as a noninvasive tool for evaluating the microvasculature in addition to the epicardial coronary arteries. Multiple studies have demonstrated that cardiac PET can detect moderate and severe angiographic CAV with high sensitivity and specificity and that abnormal results have prognostic implications. However, no study to date has shown the ability of PET to accurately detect early CAV.[15]

INVASIVE IMAGING
Coronary Angiography

The current standard of care and class I guideline-recommended modality for the surveillance and diagnosis of CAV is coronary angiography.[17] The initial description of angiographic CAV was reported by Gao and colleagues in 1998 and involved anatomic classification of lesions. The authors noted 3 distinct subtypes of angiographic CAV. Discrete, tubular, or multiple stenoses in the proximal, middle, or distal segments were coded as "type A" lesions. Diffuse concentric narrowing that began in the mid-to-distal vessel was coded as either "type B1" (abrupt onset of narrowing) or "type B2" (gradual transition with tapering). Finally, diffusely irregular vessels with loss of small branches due to nontapered and squared off terminations were designated as "type C" lesions.[18] This classification system was used for many years; however, it lacked prognostic value and ultimately fell out of favor.[19]

In 1998, a large multicenter study from the Cardiac Transplant Research Database demonstrated the prognostic implications of angiography in heart transplant recipients. Patients with angiographic evidence of CAV were found to have nearly a 20% risk of developing severe CAV within 5 years, which carried a 50% risk of death or retransplantation at 5 years.[20] In this study, angiographic CAV was categorized by the degree of primary and branch vessel stenosis, a schema that laid the foundation for the current widely used classification system. In 2010, the International Society for Heart and Lung Transplantation (ISHLT) established a

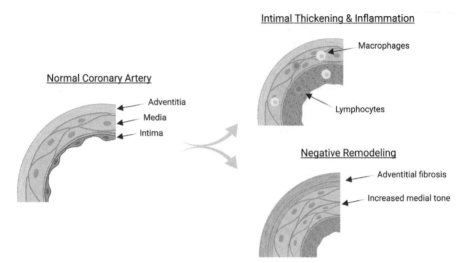

Fig. 3. Pathophysiology of CAV. Early CAV is often characterized by intimal hyperplasia owing to infiltration of inflammatory cells as well as negative remodeling due to adventitial fibrosis and increased medial tone. Over time, these dual processes result in progressive narrowing of the vessel lumen.

standardized nomenclature for grading the severity of CAV based on angiographic appearance and the presence of allograft dysfunction (left ventricular ejection fraction $\leq$45% or evidence of significant restrictive physiology). The new categories were defined as CAV_0 (not significant), CAV_1 (mild), CAV_2 (moderate), and CAV_3 (severe) (Fig. 4, Table 1).[19] Since its development, several studies have demonstrated the prognostic significance of this grading system. In one particular analysis, CAV_2 and CAV_3 were associated with greater risk of major adverse cardiovascular events (MACE) when compared with CAV_0 and CAV_1.[21]

The major strengths of angiography are its wide availability and ability to inform prognosis. However, because angiography visualizes the lumen of epicardial coronary arteries without assessing the vessel wall, it has a low sensitivity for detecting early CAV. In one study, the sensitivity and specificity of coronary angiography for detecting CAV were 42% and 95%, respectively.[22] Often, early CAV manifests as concentric luminal narrowing, and focal obstructive lesions that can be visualized by angiography do not develop until late in the disease process. For this reason, coronary angiography is commonly performed in conjunction with another intravascular imaging modality that can interrogate the vessel wall.

Intravascular Ultrasound

During the last 20 years, the use of intravascular ultrasound (IVUS) to screen for CAV has increased significantly, and it now carries a class

IIa recommendation for use in transplant recipients.[17] By providing cross-sectional imaging of the vessel wall, IVUS allows for earlier detection of intimal thickening and negative remodeling before these processes may be apparent on coronary angiography (Fig. 5). The value of IVUS for an early detection of CAV was first shown in a 1992 study comparing intimal thickness measured by IVUS to coronary angiography. The study found that, despite normal angiographic appearance, more than two-thirds of heart transplant recipients had intimal thickening by IVUS at 1 year. The authors subsequently created the Stanford classification system for grading CAV severity based on the degree of intimal thickening and circumferential extent of plaque visualized on IVUS (see Table 1).[23]

Multiple studies have since demonstrated the prognostic impact of IVUS-based parameters, namely maximal intimal thickness (MIT), in heart transplant recipients. The first study to do so used IVUS to assess 74 heart transplant recipients and found an almost 10-fold higher incidence of sudden death, myocardial infarction, or need for coronary revascularization at 4 years after transplant among patients with an MIT of greater than 0.5 mm in comparison to those with milder disease.[24] A subsequent study in 145 heart transplant patients revealed that an MIT greater than 0.3 mm was associated with decreased 4-year survival and freedom from cardiac death and retransplantation.[25] These initial studies were followed by 2 simultaneous publications in 2005 demonstrating that the progression of intimal thickening from baseline to 1 year

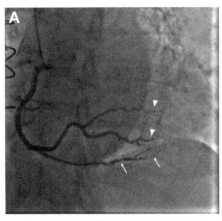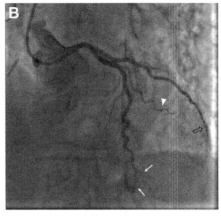

Fig. 4. Severe angiographic CAV (ISHLT CAV3). Selective coronary angiography of the right coronary system (A) demonstrates severe stenoses and distal pruning of the posterior descending (arrowheads) and posterolateral branches (arrows). Angiography of the left coronary circulation (B) also reveals severe CAV of the distal left anterior descending artery (white arrows), diagonal artery (arrowhead), and left circumflex artery (black arrow).

following transplant portended worse outcomes. In a multicenter study of 125 heart transplant patients, Kobashigawa and colleagues reported increased mortality, nonfatal MACE and angiographic CAV at 5 years among patients in whom the MIT increased by 0.5 mm or greater during the first year after transplant.[4] Similar data were published in a single-center study of 143 patients by Tuzcu and colleagues that found higher rates of mortality and a composed endpoint of death or nonfatal myocardial infarction during 6 year follow-up among those with a change in MIT of 0.5 mm or greater from baseline to 1 year.[5]

It is important to note that these seminal studies were performed before many of the current standard practices for heart transplant care were instituted. Many of the patients studied in these groundbreaking analyses were treated with cyclosporine and azathioprine as opposed to the contemporary immunosuppressive regimens favoring tacrolimus and mycophenolate. Furthermore, statins and mammalian target of rapamycin inhibitors, agents that are known to slow the progression of CAV, had not yet been widely adopted.[26] These changes and future advances in the care of heart transplant recipients may affect the validity of the aforementioned IVUS parameters for prognostication in the contemporary era. Nonetheless, data from a more recent 2015 study demonstrated that IVUS findings beyond 1 year after transplant continue to provide prognostic value. In this study, an increase in MIT by 0.35 mm or greater at 5 years after transplant was associated with an increased rate of MACE and cardiovascular mortality.[27]

For a more detailed and precise assessment of CAV by IVUS, 3-dimensional volumetric analysis can be performed to quantify early intimal thickening and negative remodeling. Many IVUS studies have revealed that negative remodeling is an integral mechanism of CAV.[6,28,29] Furthermore, evidence of negative remodeling by volumetric IVUS has also been associated with worse outcomes. For example, a study of 100 heart transplant recipients who underwent volumetric IVUS analysis found that those with negative remodeling at 1 year had greater rates of acute cellular rejection, mortality, and retransplantation during nearly 5-year follow-up.[30]

In addition to quantitative parameters, several studies have investigated qualitative IVUS findings of CAV. One such example is a study that evaluated the presence of attenuated-signal plaque (ASP), a marker of necrotic core and inflammatory plaque, and found that an episode of acute cellular rejection during the first year after transplant was associated with ASP progression at 1 year. Furthermore, patients with ASP progression had significantly higher rates of long-term mortality and retransplantation.[31] Another study reported that periarterial neovascularization on IVUS was associated with increased MIT, acute cellular rejection, and long-term mortality.[32]

Spectral analysis of IVUS radiofrequency data, also known as IVUS-virtual histology (IVUS-VH), has also been used to assess and classify plaque composition in vivo. The radiofrequency signal patterns used to identify plaque composition have been derived by performing histology of explanted vessels that were then correlated with IVUS images.[33] IVUS-VH can distinguish

Table 1
International Society for Heart and Lung Transplantation and Standford classification schemes for grading cardiac allograft vasculopathy severity

CAV Severity	ISHLT Nomenclature (Angiography-Derived)	Stanford Classification (IVUS-Derived)
Not detectable	CAV_0 • No detectable angiographic lesion • Normal allograft function by echocardiography	Class 0 • No measurable intimal layer by ultrasound
Minimal	N/A	Class I • Intimal thickness <0.3 mm • <180° extent of plaque
Mild	CAV_1 • LM < 50%, or primary vessel lesion <70%, or branch stenosis <70% • Normal allograft function by echocardiography	Class II • Intimal thickness >0.3 mm • >180° extent of plaque
Moderate	CAV_2 • LM < 50%, and single primary vessel lesion ≥70%, or isolated branch stenosis in 2 systems ≥70% • Normal allograft function by echocardiography	Class III • Intimal thickness 0.3–0.5 mm, or • > 0.5 mm and <180° extent of plaque
Severe	CAV_3 • LM ≥ 50%, or at least 2 primary vessel lesions ≥70%, or branch stenoses in all 3 systems ≥70%, or • CAV1 or CAV2 with allograft dysfunction by echocardiography	Class IV • Intimal thickness >1 mm, or • > 0.5 mm and >180° extent of plaque

Abbreviations: CAV, cardiac allograft vasculopathy; ISHLT, international society for heart and lung transplantation; IVUS, intravascular ultrasound; LM, left main.

Adapted from the 2010 ISHLT consensus statement for standardized nomenclature of CAV[19] and St Goar FG, Pinto FJ, Alderman EL, et al.[23]

plaques into 4 types: necrotic core, dense calcium, fibrous, or fibrofatty components.[34,35] In one study using IVUS-VH to assess plaque morphology among 86 heart transplant recipients in which lesions were defined as inflammatory based on the presence of necrotic core and dense calcium 30% or greater of total plaque volume, the authors observed an association between the presence of inflammatory lesions at baseline and recurrent early graft rejection and progression of CAV during 1-year follow-up.[36] Unfortunately, IVUS-VH has several limitations. Large differences between the resolution of histology and IVUS make cross-correlation between findings difficult. Furthermore, the histologic analysis from which radiofrequency signal patterns are created are neither free from artifact during the sample preparation nor free from error due to interobserver variability between pathologist interpretations.[33,34] In in vivo studies of IVUS-VH in transplanted coronary arteries, intimal thickening greater than 0.5 mm was required as a threshold for VH analysis. This threshold precludes analysis of plaque below this resolution and also limits the sensitivity of IVUS-VH for the detection of thin cap fibroatheromas, a feature of vulnerable plaque.[34–37]

Despite the fact that IVUS is the current accepted standard for early detection of CAV, it has notable limitations. Introduction of an IVUS catheter into the coronary arteries increases the risk of complications during angiography, especially if multivessel imaging is attempted. For this reason, in addition to time and cost considerations, IVUS evaluation of CAV is usually limited to assessment of the left anterior descending coronary artery. Furthermore, IVUS catheters currently on the market may be too large for imaging in smaller caliber vessels where early CAV may be most apparent. Volumetric IVUS, which provides more accurate vessel analysis, is too time-consuming for daily clinical practice. Importantly, updated studies

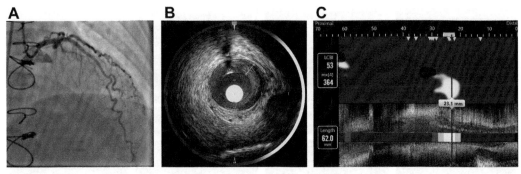

Fig. 5. Early CAV by IVUS and NIRS. Although there is no significant evidence of angiographic CAV in (*A*), intravascular imaging in this transplant recipient demonstrates significant intimal thickening of 1 mm (*blue line*) in the mid vessel on IVUS (*B*) with evidence of lipid-rich plaque by NIRS (*C*). The purple circle in panel B indicates the lumen/intima border.

evaluating the prognostic implications of IVUS parameters and cutoffs in the current era of transplant cardiology are needed.

Optical Coherence Tomography

Optical coherence tomography (OCT) is an intravascular imaging modality that uses near-infrared light to image the coronary vessel wall and was approved by the Food and Drug Administration for intracoronary use in 2010.[26,38] During the past decade, OCT is increasingly being used to optimize percutaneous coronary intervention of native coronary atherosclerosis. More recently, however, OCT has been studied in the assessment of CAV and may provide further insight into CAV pathophysiology.

Compared with IVUS, OCT offers certain technical advantages such as faster catheter pullback speeds and angiographic coregistration, although some newer IVUS platforms now have coregistration capability. One of the primary imaging advantages of OCT over IVUS is its 10-fold greater spatial resolution, which allows for visualization of intimal thickening that is less than the threshold for the detection by IVUS. Indeed, an early autopsy study comparing OCT and IVUS demonstrated superior accuracy of OCT for measuring intima-media thickness.[39] In a 2012 study of 7 heart transplant recipients, authors found that intimal hyperplasia, defined as intimal thickness greater than 100 μm, was seen in 67% of vessel segments by OCT compared with only 14% of segments by IVUS (*P* < .01). Notably, 31% of segments had intimal thickening less than 150 μm, which is less than the resolution of IVUS.[40] Another study demonstrated that OCT measurements of MIT and luminal area were noted to have lower interobserver variability than IVUS measurements.[41] In

the OCTCAV study of 15 heart transplant recipients without angiographic CAV between 1 and 4 years after transplant, Khandhar and colleagues observed a thicker intima, greater plaque volume, and greater plaque index for patients with an intima-to-media (I/M) ratio greater than 1. Although there was greater intimal and medial thickening in the proximal segment, the I/M ratio did not change throughout the analyzed portions of the vessel. The authors, therefore, proposed an I/M ratio greater than 1, as opposed to absolute values from point measurements, as a metric for defining abnormal intimal thickening by OCT.[42] More recently, three-dimensional OCT evaluation of 50 heart transplant patients revealed significant evidence of negative remodeling at 1 year after transplant.[43]

Another key strength of OCT is its ability to differentiate the plaque composition (Fig. 6). In the OCTCAV study, for example, plaque characterization was possible in all patients, including those with intimal hyperplasia. This is in contrast to VH-IVUS, where the poorer resolution of IVUS interferes with the assessment for atherosclerosis in the presence of significant intimal thickening.[42] Characterization by OCT has provided insight into the complex pathophysiology of CAV. One challenge in diagnosing CAV is distinguishing it from native and donor-derived atherosclerosis. In 2016, investigators used OCT to compare plaque morphology in 60 patients with CAV to 60 patients with native atherosclerosis. The analysis revealed that CAV was more likely to consist of diffuse and homogenous lesions, whereas lesions in native atherosclerosis were more likely to have eccentric and lipidic plaque containing calcium. Furthermore, transplant recipients with prior high-grade rejection had significantly smaller lumen area and

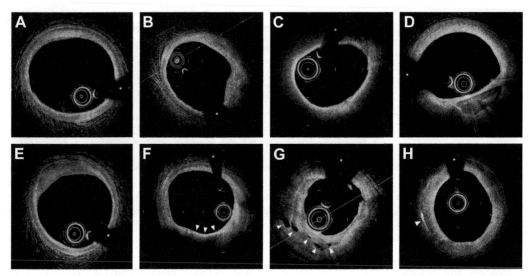

Fig. 6. Range of OCT findings in CAV. (A) Concentric fibrous intimal thickening, (B) lipid-rich plaque, (C) thin-cap fibroatheroma, (D) calcified plaque, (E) layered plaque, (F) bright spots suggesting macrophage accumulation (arrowheads), (G) microvessels in intima (arrowheads), (H) cholesterol crystal (arrowhead). Asterisk indicates Guidewire artifact.

greater macrophage infiltration than those with native atherosclerosis.[44] Interestingly, when investigators from the Mayo Clinic used OCT to characterize CAV lesions in 53 heart transplant recipients, they found a significantly higher prevalence of lesions with findings of typical atherosclerosis (eg, eccentric plaque with lipid pools and calcification) as time from transplant increased. Furthermore, the presence vulnerable plaque (defined by features such as thin-cap fibroatheroma, macrophages, and microchannels) and complex lesions (containing intimal laceration, intraluminal thrombus, and layered complex plaque) also increased substantially with time from transplantation.[45] The association of neovascularization and microchannels with intimal thickening and the presence of CAV has been confirmed in subsequent studies.[46,47] Another study similarly found that lipid pools, thin-cap fibroatheroma, macrophages, and microchannels identified on OCT at baseline were predictive of CAV progression on IVUS at 1 year.[48]

Despite its many strengths, there are key limitations of OCT use that should be considered. Imaging with OCT requires additional contrast administration for coronary flushing, which may be prohibitive in transplant recipients that have renal dysfunction. Additionally, OCT has a lower tissue penetration than IVUS, which may limit delineation of the intima-media interface and preclude assessment of plaque burden when intimal thickness exceeds 1.5 mm or in the setting of a thick fibrous cap.[49] Finally, and

perhaps most importantly, there are no studies to date establishing the prognostic significance of OCT-based parameters as there are with IVUS. Further studies are needed to determine which OCT parameters and plaque components are associated with adverse clinical outcomes before OCT is endorsed by societal guidelines for CAV screening. These studies may also shed further light on the pathophysiology of CAV, risk factors associated with its development and progression, and potential targets for novel therapeutics.

Near-Infrared Spectroscopy

Near-infrared spectroscopy (NIRS) is the most recent addition to the invasive imaging armamentarium. Intracoronary NIRS identifies the presence of lipid-rich plaque by generating a unique chemogram, or color map, that denotes the distribution of the probability of lipid-rich plaque on a color scale from red to yellow (see Fig. 5).[50] Autopsy studies have validated the chemical pattern of lipid-rich plaque detected by NIRS.[51] The amount of lipid in a vessel segment is quantified on a scale of 0 to 1000 to measure the lipid core burden index (LCBI), which is typically reported as the maximum LCBI within a 4 mm segment.[50,52] Since its introduction, NIRS has been combined with IVUS into one imaging catheter platform, and its use for identifying vulnerable plaque in native atherosclerosis has been increasingly studied.[53–55] However, few studies have been conducted to

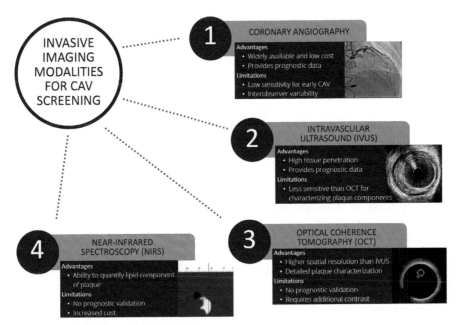

Fig. 7. Comparison of invasive imaging modalities for CAV screening.

assess the benefits of NIRS in the heart transplant population.

In an early application of NIRS for the assessment of CAV, investigators compared the chemograms of 2 transplant recipients with different survival times. They observed predominantly fibrotic plaque in the patient with the more recent transplant history, as opposed to lipid-rich plaque in the patient with an older allograft (52). More recently, a larger study used NIRS to compare CAV in 28 heart transplant patients with native atherosclerosis in 27 nontransplant patients and showed that transplant patients had a greater maxLCBI$_{4mm}$ than patients with native atherosclerosis in vessel segments with similarly mild plaque burden, suggesting that CAV may involve more accelerated lipid accumulation.[50] These data are consistent with earlier findings from a smaller study in which 83% of heart transplant patients imaged with NIRS early after transplant had lipidic plaque.[56] NIRS has also been used to demonstrate an association between lipid accumulation in plaque and a history of acute rejection; specifically, a maxLCBI$_{4mm}$ greater than 200 had a sensitivity of 62% and specificity of 85% for identifying patients with a history of high-grade acute rejection.[57]

Despite these intriguing preliminary data, a few limitations of NIRS are worth noting. First, although NIRS has excellent sensitivity for detecting lipid-rich plaque, it has poor depth resolution. Second, as with OCT, there are no

published prognostic data to date for LCBI in CAV. However, the combined NIRS-IVUS imaging platform should facilitate adoption by operators who are already competent and comfortable with performing IVUS, and in turn accelerate outcome studies of NIRS in the heart transplant population.

FUTURE DIRECTIONS

Ongoing development of emerging invasive intracoronary imaging technologies is underway, paving the way for additional potential tools to diagnose CAV earlier and better understand its pathophysiology. One such example is near-infrared autofluorescence, which identifies vulnerable plaque by detecting elevated levels of autofluorescence emitted by a lipid-rich plaque with necrotic core.[58] In addition to new modalities, intracoronary imaging platforms are now being combined into hybrid imaging systems (eg, NIRS-IVUS), allowing for simultaneous anatomic and compositional analysis of lesions. This strategy may also lead to wider adoption of these emerging technologies. Examples of up-and-coming combined imaging platforms include OCT-NIRS (SpectraWave, Bedford, MA, USA), OCT-IVUS (Terumo, Tokyo, Japan and Conavi Medical Inc., Toronto, Canada), and OCT-NIRAF (recently developed by the Tearney Lab at Harvard Medical School) (58).

Importantly, studies using invasive intracoronary imaging to assess the efficacy of alternative immunosuppressive strategies and the role of potential new preventive therapies for CAV are currently underway. For example, the AERIAL trial (NCT04770012) will use OCT to investigate whether early antiplatelet therapy prevents the development of CAV. Additional ongoing trials include the use of OCT and IVUS to determine the efficacy of proprotein convertase subtilisin/kexin type 9 inhibitors for CAV prevention (NCT04193306 and NCT03734211).

SUMMARY

CAV is a leading cause of long-term mortality among heart transplant recipients. The prevention, early diagnosis, and treatment of CAV are imperative for improving outcomes and increasing survival. Although coronary angiography is the established standard for CAV screening, IVUS has more or less supplanted angiography in the contemporary era through its ability to detect early CAV and provide prognostic data. Additional technologies such as OCT and NIRS that offer further mechanistic insights into CAV are emerging in this space, although outcome data are needed before they are incorporated into societal guidelines and the current CAV surveillance paradigm. Although there are important strengths and weaknesses for each imaging technology (Fig. 7), hybrid platforms have the potential to mitigate these limitations and provide complementary data. Ongoing outcome studies may validate these newer invasive intracoronary imaging modalities for prognostication in heart transplant recipients and shed light on potential novel therapeutic targets and agents.

CLINICS CARE POINTS

- Noninvasive imaging modalities suffer from poor sensitivity for detecting early CAV, therefore making routine invasive intravascular imaging essential in the early posttransplant course.

- Coronary angiography and IVUS provide valuable prognostic information in heart transplant recipients.

- Newer invasive intracoronary imaging modalities such as OCT and NIRS are elucidating important pathophysiologic mechanisms of CAV but have yet to demonstrate an association with outcomes in the heart transplant population.

ACKNOWLEDGMENTS

The authors thank Kan Saito for his assistance in creating Fig. 6.

DISCLOSURE

R.V. Parikh receives research support from the American Heart Association, United States, Janssen, United States, InfraRedx, United States, and Abbott Vascular, United States, unrelated research support from Bayer, Germany, and unrelated consulting fees from Abbott Vascular. N. Shahandeh reports no relationships with industry relevant to the contents of this article to disclose.

REFERENCES

1. Cooper DK. Christiaan Barnard and his contributions to heart transplantation. J Heart Lung Transpl 2001;20(6):599–610.
2. Khush KK, Cherikh WS, Chambers DC, et al. The international thoracic organ transplant registry of the international society for heart and lung transplantation: thirty-sixth adult heart transplantation report - 2019; focus theme: donor and recipient size match. J Heart Lung Transpl 2019;38(10):1056–66.
3. Lund LH, Edwards LB, Kucheryavaya AY, et al. The Registry of the International Society for Heart and Lung Transplantation: Thirty-second Official Adult Heart Transplant Report–2015; Focus Theme: Early Graft Failure. J Heart Lung Transpl Off. Publ. Int. Soc. Heart Transpl 2015;34:1244–54.
4. Kobashigawa JA, Tobis JM, Starling RC, et al. Multicenter intravascular ultrasound validation study among heart transplant recipients: outcomes after five years. J Am Coll Cardiol 2005; 45:1532–7.
5. Tuzcu EM, Kapadia SR, Sachar R, et al. Intravascular ultrasound evidence of angiographically silent progression in coronary atherosclerosis predicts long-term morbidity and mortality after cardiac transplantation. J Am Coll Cardiol 2005;45:1538–42.
6. Mitchell RN, Libby P. Vascular remodeling in transplant vasculopathy. Circ Res 2007;100:967–78.
7. ISHLT 2019 Registry Report. J Heart Lung Transpl 2019;38(10):1015–66.
8. Pollack A, Nazif T, Mancini D, et al. Detection and imaging of cardiac allograft vasculopathy. JACC: Cardiovasc Imaging 2013;6(5):613–23.
9. Chih S, Chong AY, Mielniczuk LM, et al. Allograft Vasculopathy: The Achilles' Heel of Heart Transplantation. J Am Coll Cardiol 2016;68:80–91.
10. Nikolova AP, Kobashigawa JA. Cardiac allograft vasculopathy: the enduring enemy of cardiac transplantation. Transplantation 2019;103(7):1338–48.
11. Lee F, Nair V, Chih S. Cardiac allograft vasculopathy: Insights on pathogenesis and therapy. Clin Transpl 2020;34(3):e13794.

12. Ciliberto GR, Ruffini L, Mangiavacchi M, et al. Resting echocardiography and quantitative dipyridamole technetium-99m sestamibi tomography in the identification of cardiac allograft vasculopathy and the prediction of long-term prognosis after heart transplantation. Eur Heart J 2001;22(11): 964–71.

13. Spes CH, Klauss V, Mudra H, et al. Diagnostic and prognostic value of serial dobutamine stress echocardiography for noninvasive assessment of cardiac allograft vasculopathy: a comparison with coronary angiography and intravascular ultrasound. Circulation 1999;100(5):509–15.

14. Wever-Pinzon O, Romero J, Kelesidis I, et al. Coronary computed tomography angiography for the detection of cardiac allograft vasculopathy: a meta-analysis of prospective trials. J Am Coll Cardiol 2014;63(19):1992–2004.

15. Madamanchi C, Konerman MC, Murthy VL. Imaging Coronary Allograft Vasculopathy with Cardiac PET and Cardiac MRI. Curr Cardiol Rep 2021; 23(12):175.

16. Chirakarnjanakorn S, Starling RC, Popović ZB, et al. Dobutamine stress echocardiography during follow-up surveillance in heart transplant patients: Diagnostic accuracy and predictors of outcomes. J Heart Lung Transpl 2015;34(5):710–7.

17. Costanzo MR, Dipchand A, Starling R, et al. The international society of heart and lung transplantation guidelines for the care of heart transplant recipients. J Heart Lung Transpl 2010;29(8):914–56.

18. Gao SZ, Alderman EL, Schroeder JS, et al. Accelerated coronary vascular disease in the heart transplant patient: coronary arteriographic findings. J Am Coll Cardiol 1988;12(2):334–40.

19. Mehra MR, Crespo-Leiro MG, Dipchand A, et al. International Society for Heart and Lung Transplantation working formulation of a standardized nomenclature for cardiac allograft vasculopathy—2010. The J Heart Lung Transplant 2010;29(7): 717–27.

20. Costanzo MR, Naftel DC, Pritzker MR, et al. Heart transplant coronary artery disease detected by coronary angiography: a multiinstitutional study of preoperative donor and recipient risk factors. Cardiac Transplant Research Database. J Heart Lung Transpl 1998;17(8):744–53.

21. Prada-Delgado O, Estévez-Loureiro R, Paniagua-Martín MJ, et al. Prevalence and prognostic value of cardiac allograft vasculopathy 1 year after heart transplantation according to the ISHLT recommended nomenclature. J Heart Lung Transpl 2012; 31(3):332–3.

22. Tuzcu EM, Hobbs RE, Rincon G, et al. Occult and frequent transmission of atherosclerotic coronary disease with cardiac transplantation. Insights from intravascular ultrasound. Circulation 1995;91(6): 1706–13.

23. St Goar FG, Pinto FJ, Alderman EL, et al. Intracoronary ultrasound in cardiac transplant recipients. In vivo evidence of "angiographically silent" intimal thickening. Circulation 1992;85(3):979–87.

24. Mehra MR, Ventura HO, Stapleton DD, et al. Presence of severe intimal thickening by intravascular ultrasonography predicts cardiac events in cardiac allograft vasculopathy. J Heart Lung Transpl 1995; 14(4):632–9.

25. Rickenbacher PR, Pinto FJ, Lewis NP, et al. Prognostic importance of intimal thickness as measured by intracoronary ultrasound after cardiac transplantation. Circulation 1995;92(12):3445–52.

26. Olymbios M, Kwiecinski J, Berman DS, et al. Imaging in heart transplant patients. JACC Cardiovasc Imaging 2018;11(10):1514–30.

27. Potena L, Masetti M, Sabatino M, et al. Interplay of coronary angiography and intravascular ultrasound in predicting long-term outcomes after heart transplantation. J Heart Lung Transpl 2015;34(9):1146–53.

28. Kobashigawa J, Wener L, Johnson J, et al. Longitudinal study of vascular remodeling in coronary arteries after heart transplantation. J Heart Lung Transpl 2000;19(6):546–50.

29. Tsutsui H, Ziada KM, Schoenhagen P, et al. Lumen loss in transplant coronary artery disease is a biphasic process involving early intimal thickening and late constrictive remodeling: results from a 5-year serial intravascular ultrasound study. Circulation 2001;104(6):653–7.

30. Okada K, Kitahara H, Yang H-M, et al. Paradoxical vessel remodeling of the proximal segment of the left anterior descending artery predicts long-term mortality after heart transplantation. JACC Heart Fail 2015;3(12):942–52.

31. Okada K, Fearon WF, Luikart H, et al. Attenuated-signal plaque progression predicts long-term mortality after heart transplantation: IVUS assessment of cardiac allograft vasculopathy. J Am Coll Cardiol 2016;68(4):382–92.

32. Kitahara H, Okada K, Tanaka S, et al. Association of periarterial neovascularization with progression of cardiac allograft vasculopathy and long-term clinical outcomes in heart transplant recipients. J Heart Lung Transpl 2016;35(6):752–9.

33. Garcìa-Garcìa HM, Gogas BD, Serruys PW, et al. IVUS-based imaging modalities for tissue characterization: similarities and differences. Int J Cardiovasc Imaging 2011;27(2):215–24.

34. Nair A, Kuban BD, Tuzcu EM, et al. Coronary plaque classification with intravascular ultrasound radiofrequency data analysis. Circulation 2002; 106(17):2200–6.

35. Nasu K, Tsuchikane E, Katoh O, et al. Accuracy of in vivo coronary plaque morphology assessment: a validation study of in vivo virtual histology compared with in vitro histopathology. J Am Coll Cardiol 2006;47(12):2405–12.

36. Raichlin E, Bae J-H, Kushwaha SS, et al. Inflammatory burden of cardiac allograft coronary atherosclerotic plaque is associated with early recurrent cellular rejection and predicts a higher risk of vasculopathy progression. J Am Coll Cardiol 2009; 53(15):1279–86.

37. Hernandez JM, de Prada JAV, Burgos V, et al. Virtual histology intravascular ultrasound assessment of cardiac allograft vasculopathy from 1 to 20 years after heart transplantation. J Heart Lung Transplant 2009;28(2):156–62.

38. Acharya D, Loyaga-Rendon RY, Chatterjee A, et al. Optical Coherence Tomography in Cardiac Allograft Vasculopathy: State-of-the-Art Review. Circ Heart Fail 2021;14(9):e008416.

39. Kume T, Akasaka T, Kawamoto T, et al. Assessment of coronary intima–media thickness by optical coherence tomography: comparison with intravascular ultrasound. Circ J 2005 Aug;69(8):903–7.

40. Hou J, Lv H, Jia H, et al. OCT assessment of allograft vasculopathy in heart transplant recipients. JACC Cardiovasc Imaging 2012;5(6):662–3.

41. Garrido IP, García-Lara J, Pinar E, et al. Optical coherence tomography and highly sensitivity troponin T for evaluating cardiac allograft vasculopathy. Am J Cardiol 2012;110(5):655–61.

42. Khandhar SJ, Yamamoto H, Teuteberg JJ, et al. Optical coherence tomography for characterization of cardiac allograft vasculopathy after heart transplantation (OCTCAV study). J Heart Lung Transpl 2013;32(6):596–602.

43. Pazdernik M, Chen Z, Bedanova H, et al. Early detection of cardiac allograft vasculopathy using highly automated 3-dimensional optical coherence tomography analysis. J Heart Lung Transpl 2018; 37(8):992–1000.

44. Shan P, Dong L, Maehara A, et al. Comparison Between Cardiac Allograft Vasculopathy and Native Coronary Atherosclerosis by Optical Coherence Tomography. Am J Cardiol 2016 Apr 15;117(8):1361–8.

45. Cassar A, Matsuo Y, Herrmann J, et al. Coronary atherosclerosis with vulnerable plaque and complicated lesions in transplant recipients: new insight into cardiac allograft vasculopathy by optical coherence tomography. Eur Heart J 2013;34(33):2610–7.

46. Ichibori Y, Ohtani T, Nakatani D, et al. Optical coherence tomography and intravascular ultrasound evaluation of cardiac allograft vasculopathy with and without intimal neovascularization. Eur Heart J Cardiovasc Imaging 2016;17(1):51–8.

47. Chahal DS, Parikh R, Yoo D, et al. Association of intimal neovessels noted by optical coherence tomography with cardiac allograft vasculopathy. Cureus 2020;12(3):e7454.

48. Park K-H, Sun T, Liu Z, et al. Relationship between markers of plaque vulnerability in optical coherence tomography and atherosclerotic progression in adult patients with heart transplantation. J Heart Lung Transpl 2017;36(2):185–92.

49. Manfrini O, Mont E, Leone O, et al. Sources of error and interpretation of plaque morphology by optical coherence tomography. Am J Cardiol 2006; 98(2):156–9.

50. Zheng B, Maehara A, Mintz GS, et al. In vivo comparison between cardiac allograft vasculopathy and native atherosclerosis using near-infrared spectroscopy and intravascular ultrasound. Eur Heart J Cardiovasc Imaging 2015;16(9):985–91.

51. Waxman S, Dixon SR, L'Allier P, et al. In vivo validation of a catheter-based near-infrared spectroscopy system for detection of lipid core coronary plaques: initial results of the SPECTACL study. JACC Cardiovasc Imaging 2009;2(7):858–68.

52. Sharma R, Roleder T, Ali Z, et al. Lipid-rich versus fibrous intimal hyperplasia in transplant vasculopathy. JACC Cardiovasc Imaging 2013;6(1):126–7.

53. Goldstein JA, Maini B, Dixon SR, et al. Detection of lipid-core plaques by intracoronary near-infrared spectroscopy identifies high risk of periprocedural myocardial infarction. Circ Cardiovasc Interv 2011; 4(5):429–37.

54. Madder RD, Goldstein JA, Madden SP, et al. Detection by near-infrared spectroscopy of large lipid core plaques at culprit sites in patients with acute ST-segment elevation myocardial infarction. JACC Cardiovasc Interv 2013;6(8):838–46.

55. Waksman R, Di Mario C, Torguson R, et al. Identification of patients and plaques vulnerable to future coronary events with near-infrared spectroscopy intravascular ultrasound imaging: a prospective, cohort study. Lancet 2019;394(10209):1629–37.

56. Cheng RK, Bhutani S, Gevorgyan R, et al. Quantification of lipid burden in heart transplant (HT) patients by near-infrared spectroscopy (NIRS). J Heart Lung Transplant 2013;32(4):S209.

57. Zheng B, Maehara A, Mintz GS, et al. Increased coronary lipid accumulation in heart transplant recipients with prior high-grade cellular rejection: novel insights from near-infrared spectroscopy. Int J Cardiovasc Imaging 2016;32(2):225–34.

58. Ughi GJ, Wang H, Gerbaud E, et al. Clinical Characterization of Coronary Atherosclerosis With Dual-Modality OCT and Near-Infrared Autofluorescence Imaging. JACC Cardiovasc Imaging 2016 Nov;9(11):1304–14.

Clinical Implication and Optimal Management of Myocardial Bridging: Role of Cardiovascular Imaging

Takehiro Hashikata, MD*, Ryo Kameda, MD,
Junya Ako, MD

KEYWORDS

- Myocardial bridge • Ischemia with no obstructive coronary arteries • Intravascular ultrasound
- Coronary computed tomography angiography • Surgical unroofing

---

KEY POINTS

- Although common in general population, the presence of a myocardial bridging (MB) is a potential cause of ischemic symptoms and adverse cardiac events.
- The clinical implication of an MB can be estimated by plaque progression upstream of the MB, the extent and degree of systolic vessel compression, and vessel restriction during diastole, as assessed using intravascular ultrasound and/or coronary computed tomography angiography.
- Optimal management by medical therapy or surgical unroofing should be considered in MB patients with refractory angina.

INTRODUCTION

Ischemia with no obstructive coronary arteries (INOCA) is a commonly recognized concept but poorly understood. Approximately half of the patients undergoing coronary angiography concerning chest pain are found to have no obstructive coronary artery disease (CAD).[1,2] Physicians often struggle to provide optimal diagnosis and management for these patients because of a lack of universal guidance. Several studies have verified epicardial endothelial or microvascular dysfunction as a cause of angina, but quite a few patients show no such dysfunctions at testing.[3-5] Although these patients may have a noncardiac etiology for their chest pain, the prevalence of myocardial bridging (MB) in this cohort was reported to be over double or triple compared with general population, which may partly account for the angina of unknown cause.[3,6]

An MB is an anatomic variant in which a portion of a coronary artery is covered by a myocardium band, located commonly in the midportion of the left anterior descending artery (LAD).[7-10] MB was historically considered a benign structure because arterial compression by MB alters blood flow primarily in systole while coronary flow in the LAD occurs predominantly during the diastolic phase of each cardiac cycle. Owing to the preserved perfusion in diastole, the majority of people with MB are indeed asymptomatic. Importantly, however, multiple recent studies have shown that MB can disrupt coronary perfusion during the whole cardiac cycle, resulting in that a certain subset of patients with MB may present with ischemic symptoms including angina, myocardial infarction, conduction disturbances, or sudden death.[11-16] In clinical practice, accurate identification of high-risk MB patients susceptible to these complications is crucial as it helps determine the strategy of

---

Department of Cardiovascular Medicine, Kitasato University School of Medicine, Kanagawa, Japan
* Corresponding author. Kitasato University School of Medicine, 1-15-1 Kitasato, Sagamihara, Kanagawa 252-0373, Japan.
E-mail address: t_hashikata@med.kitasato-u.ac.jp

Intervent Cardiol Clin 12 (2023) 281–288
https://doi.org/10.1016/j.iccl.2022.12.007

management and therapeutic approaches in addition to providing prognostic information. Hence, the present review summarizes the clinical implication and management of MB, highlighting the role of imaging modalities currently available in this arena.

PREVALENCE OF MYOCARDIAL BRIDGING

The true prevalence of MB has not been fully elucidated and it depends largely on the evaluation modalities, populations investigated, and physician's experience. It is also known that the use of medication such as nitroglycerin or dobutamine augments the degree of arterial compression by MB.[17,18] The frequency of an MB was reported as 0.5% to 33% of cases assessed by coronary angiography,[9,19–21] 23% by intravascular ultrasound (IVUS),[22] 25% to 30% by coronary computed tomography angiography (CCTA),[23–25] and up to 85% in autopsy series.[26] In addition to the varying study populations, the wide range of those reported rates is likely attributed to the different sensitivity for the detection of an MB in each modality. As of today, IVUS is considered to offer the most detailed anatomical and dynamic assessment of an MB by its performance, providing 70 to 200-μm axial-resolution real-time images (with a center transducer frequency of 20 to 60 MHz) and precise geographic assessment including a relationship with the LAD and involved branches. MB is dominantly located in LAD in 70% to 98% of cases, whereas it is also found infrequently in left circumflex and right coronary arteries.[25,27,28]

CLINICAL SIGNIFICANCE OF MYOCARDIAL BRIDGING

According to the clinical reports using IVUS and/or CCTA examination, at least one-fourth of overall populations may have a clinically identifiable MB regardless of its significance. Because of this relatively high frequency as well as the false recognition that systolic arterial compression by MB would not affect myocardial perfusion occurring primarily in diastole, the clinical significance of MB is often underestimated in daily practice worldwide. Although multiple studies have indicated that the presence of an MB can cause angina and/or poor clinical outcomes in a subset of patients,[11–16] such patients often receive conventional management as an INOCA due to spasm, endothelial dysfunction (ie, syndrome X), or an unknown cause without undergoing further hemodynamic and vascular imaging assessments.

The adverse effects of MB likely result from several specific mechanisms: (1) acceleration of atherosclerotic plaque upstream from MB, (2) delayed coronary arterial relaxation in diastole, (3) high frequency of endothelial dysfunction, and (4) persistent diastolic structural restriction of the tunneled segment.

Previous autopsy,[8,29] angiographic,[22] and CCTA,[30] and IVUS[31] studies showed a greater plaque burden in the LAD segment proximal to the MB than within the tunneled LAD segment. The anatomic significance of an MB, such as its greater length, thickness, and systolic compression by MB can accelerate atherosclerotic plaque formation located proximally to MBs despite having low risks of CAD, which possibly leads to unexpected adverse cardiovascular events.[31,32] Yamada and colleagues[33] showed that the extent of plaque progression 20 mm proximal to a bridged segment, as assessed by IVUS, related to the degree of systolic compression within the MB segment. This preferential location of MB-related atherosclerotic plaque may be in part associated with hemodynamic disturbances caused by cyclic muscle contraction of MB. Notably, the distribution of wall shear stress related to the tunneled segment is important as low shear stress is known to enhance lipid transfer across the endothelium, resulting in atherosclerotic plaque formation localized in such segments. A report using a computational fluid dynamics model of the LAD in a symptomatic MB patient showed lower wall shear stress proximal and distal to the MB compared with the tunneled segment.[34] A case-control study of MB patients also showed that the wall shear rate, the velocity gradient perpendicular to the wall, was lower in the segment proximal to the MB than within the tunneled segment.[35] Other potential mechanisms for proximal plaque formation include abnormal flow profiles at this segment such as oscillatory flow reversal against the antegrade coronary flow. Several studies have revealed that arterial segments in which blood flow departs from a laminar unidirectional pattern may lead to the development of plaque formation.[36–38]

It is well known that coronary blood flow in the LAD predominantly occurs during the diastolic phase of the cardiac cycle, and therefore, it appears likely that arterial compression in the systolic phase could not significantly impact myocardial perfusion by itself. Delayed opening of the coronary artery after the systolic compression by MB can rather contribute to the development of myocardial ischemia because of insufficient inflow time, resulting in hemodynamic disturbances.[39–43] Lin and colleagues[11] showed that change in the blood perfusion from delayed arterial relaxation in diastole or the Venturi effect on the septal branches by MB may cause functional ischemia in the affected myocardial perfusion territory. Other occult coronary abnormalities, in particular the endothelial dysfunction, are frequently present in the tunneled artery, which can trigger coronary vasospasm and platelet aggregation resulting in acute coronary syndrome in a clinical setting.[44,45] Other studies also showed that endothelial dysfunction assessed by acetylcholine testing was observed in over 85% of patients with significant MB, and 23% had microvascular dysfunction defined as the index of microcirculatory resistance ≥ 25.[18,46]

Although the severity of an MB is often estimated by the extent and degree of systolic vessel compression or angiographic "milking" in clinical practice, Hashikata and colleagues[16] first revealed the importance of MB assessment in diastole as well. Out of 111 patients with refractory angina despite maximally tolerated medical management, 97 patients (87%) had persistent diastolic vessel structural reduction in end-diastole or "diastolic vessel restriction" within the MB segment; greater diastolic vessel restriction was significantly associated with the degree of limiting their quality of life. As described above, coronary blood flow in the LAD primarily occurs during the diastolic phase of the cardiac cycle. In the presence of a flow disturbance in systole by vessel compression, effective antegrade blood perfusion may depend almost exclusively on the diastolic coronary flow, though the flow in diastole can be diminished with delayed or restricted arterial relaxation caused by the overlying MB.[43,47] The angina symptoms caused by this mechanism can be further exacerbated with the shortening of diastole in tachycardia during stress or exercise in daily activities.

EVALUATION OF PATIENTS WITH SUSPECTED MYOCARDIAL BRIDGING
Noninvasive Stress Echocardiography
Patients with angina generally undergo some sort of noninvasive stress testing as an initial evaluation to screen for obstructive or no obstructive CAD. Stress echocardiography and stress nuclear myocardial perfusion imaging have been historically used and found to have relatively good accuracy. The typical finding on these tests suggesting a significant fixed obstructive coronary lesion is the presence of an inducible regional wall motion abnormality or inducible perfusion defect. On the other hand, the utility of these tests had not been well validated in patients with occult coronary abnormality such as endothelial dysfunction and microvascular dysfunction.[48] In 2013, an echocardiographic pattern of focal end-systolic to early-diastolic buckling in the septum with apical sparing was reported in a series of symptomatic patients with LAD MB,[11] potentially serving as a characteristic finding for diagnosis of clinically significant MB with a noninvasive stress test. Pargaonkar and colleagues[49] subsequently showed that the presence of "focal septal buckling with apical sparing" on stress echocardiography had a sensitivity of 90% and a specificity of 83% for identifying an MB as referenced to CCTA, as well as a positive predictive value of 97% and a negative predictive value of 63%, albeit in a small cohort of patients (n = 37).

Coronary Computed Tomography Angiography
Noninvasive CCTA is recently preferred as the initial examination to evaluate patients who present with typical or atypical chest pain due to its high accuracy of assessment for the presence, extent, and severity of CAD.[50,51] As expected, CCTA can provide relatively accurate anatomical assessments of overlying MB as well as intracoronary plaque and structural information of vessels. CCTA has been used as a reference standard for the presence or absence of an MB, and also to discern no obstructive CAD.[49,52] The vessel encasement by MB can be graded on CCTA findings: partial encasement, defined as the vessel within the interventricular groove and in direct contact with the left ventricular myocardium (Grade 1), and full encasement, defined as the vessel surrounded by the myocardium without (Grade 2) or with (Grade 3) measurable overlying muscle.[52] Compared with IVUS, lower spatial resolution of CCTA may result in a slight underestimation of MB length (approximately -2.0 mm on average) due to the difference in the determination of the entrance and exit of the MB segment. Nevertheless, the anatomical assessment of MB by CCTA, such as its length and depth, generally have reasonable agreements with those of IVUS. In MB patients with refractory angina, Hashikata and colleagues[16] showed a significant correlation in total MB length between the two modalities ($P < .0001$, $R^2 = 0.61$). A greater degree of the CCTA grade was also associated with a greater halo thickness or MB depth measured by IVUS (0.44 ± 0.05 mm in Grade 1, 0.66 ± 0.05 mm in Grade 2, and 1.02 ± 0.05 mm in Grade 3).

Invasive Coronary Angiography

On coronary angiography, visual interpretation of an MB is commonly made based on systolic compression of an intramyocardial portion of a coronary artery (ie, milking effect). In other words, physicians typically distinguish bridging from other types of coronary abnormalities by observing the phase-dependent dynamic obstruction. MBs are often associated with the presence of endothelial dysfunction,[18,46] and the use of nitroglycerin augments the severity of the compression by an MB.[17,43] Hence, acetylcholine testing and intracoronary nitroglycerin infusion should be conducted with detailed MB assessments. Of note, however, contrast angiography is the least sensitive imaging, as an MB can be diagnosed only indirectly by detecting systolic squeezing.[9,22] Symptomatic patients suggestive of a substantial LAD MB on CCTA or angiography should go on to have detailed IVUS and hemodynamic assessments to judge the significance of the MB (Fig. 1).

Intracoronary Imaging

Currently, IVUS is considered the gold standard for the anatomic assessment of MBs as it can directly visualize the vessel wall and perivascular structures at a high resolution and in real time, enabling a precise and dynamic assessment of an MB and the tunneled coronary artery. Standard anatomical MB characteristics assessable by IVUS include the location, length, thickness, degree of systolic arterial compression as a dynamic property, and the number of septal and diagonal branches originating within the tunneled arterial segment (Fig. 2). The characteristic appearance is a "half-moon" sign, representing an echo-lucent area present in the perivascular space immediately adjacent to the coronary artery that persists throughout the cardiac cycle. Compared with CCTA and optical coherence tomography (OCT), IVUS with slow automated pullback (0.5 mm/s recommended) allows dynamic assessment of an MB and the affected coronary artery. Pargaonkar and colleagues[18] reported that the MB muscle index (the total MB length × halo thickness) assessed by IVUS can be used to identify the hemodynamic significance of an MB.

OCT may also be used as a higher-resolution intravascular imaging technology for MB assessment. On OCT, MB can be visualized as an intermediate optical intensity, fine layer surrounding the coronary artery.[53,54] However, its limited imaging depth may preclude the whole visualization of an MB beyond the artery, and more importantly, the dynamic MB assessment related to the cardiac cycle is not possible with the ultra-fast pullback of OCT for blood washout. Despite these technical limitations, OCT may offer some unique information by its microscopic resolution, such as the evaluation of adventitial vasa vasorum.[54,55] The vasa vasorum plays a significant role as a source of various inflammatory mediators resulting in the growth of atherosclerosis and coronary spasm, and a small OCT series of MB patients showed the absence of adventitial vasa vasorum at the MB segment with its increased formation at the proximal references.[54] Combined together, a novel IVUS-OCT hybrid system may work synergistically and facilitate a greater understanding of pathophysiology as well as a comprehensive clinical assessment of MBs.

TREATMENT OF SYMPTOMATIC MYOCARDIAL BRIDGING

To date, there are no established guidelines for the treatment of QOL-limiting symptomatic MBs, particularly for patients with refractory angina against optimal medical therapy. Medical therapy primarily consists of beta-blockers and nondihydropyridine calcium-channel blockers. Beta-blockers can reduce vessel compression by the muscular band as well as the heart rate resulting in a prolonged diastolic period.[42,56] Nondihydropyridine calcium channel blockers can be helpful to improve endothelial dysfunction and reduce the compression of the artery.[57] In contrast, vasodilators, such as nitrates, have been considered a contraindication in MB patients, shown to accentuate systolic compression of the MB segment, and indeed is often used as an agent for provocation of this phenomenon.[10]

Stent placement, in theory, can directly improve both the systolic compression and diastolic restriction within the MB segment by reinforcing the intramural coronary artery. However, controversy remains due to potential complications, such as coronary perforation, coronary spasm, stent strut fracture, and in-stent restenosis, derived from mechanical interaction between the permanently implanted device and MB.[58,59] Although coronary artery bypass has been performed as a surgical treatment strategy for symptomatic MB, the result of the surgery has not been satisfactory (ie, frequent graft occlusion), especially using an internal mammary artery graft than a saphenous vein graft.[60,61] Contrary to these conventional invasive treatments with controversial results, surgical unroofing, or supra-arterial myotomy of an MB, may better address the MB pathologies and has

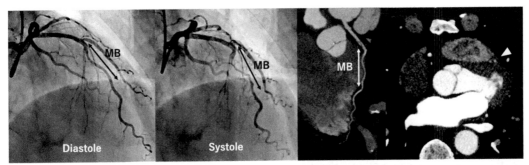

Fig. 1. Coronary angiography and CCTA findings of MB. Coronary angiography shows typical arterial compression in systole and vessel restriction even in diastole in the middle segment of the LAD. On CCTA, full encasement of the LAD by the myocardium with measurable overlying muscle (*arrowhead*) is observed at the corresponding segment (Grade 3).

been attempted in symptomatic MB patients with excellent mid and long-term outcomes reported since 1975. Single-center experience mounting at Stanford University in both adults and pediatrics has also shown significant improvements in quality of life after surgical unroofing without any major complications or death.[62–64] Further research is warranted to investigate whether the effect of surgical unroofing is applicable to improvement in MB-related hard endpoints as well, such as myocardial infarction, conduction disturbances, or sudden cardiac death. Of note, epicardial adipose tissue overlying the LAD artery usually precludes

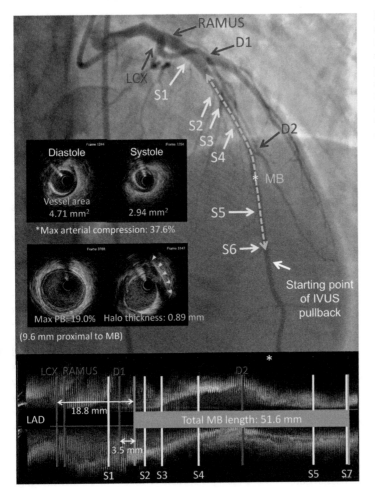

Fig. 2. Example of systematic anatomical MB assessment with IVUS: IVUS-MAP. IVUS transducer was placed as far distally as safely possible in the LAD, followed by image acquisition performed with automated pullback at 0.5 mm/s (recommended). An MB was identified as an echolucent half-moon sign (halo) lying on top of the artery (*blue arrowheads*). In addition to its morphologic characteristics, total MB length, halo thickness, and a degree of arterial compression were measured. Maximum plaque burden (Max PB) upstream of MB and number of septal (S) and diagonal (D) branches originating within the tunneled arterial segment were also evaluated. The arterial compression was calculated as (diastolic vessel area–systolic vessel area)/diastolic vessel area × 100 at maximum compression site (*). This systematic assessment is summarized as an "IVUS-MAP" of the LAD MB. In this particular example, the MB was observed between the first and sixth septal perforators with a landmark of the second diagonal branch originating from the center of the tunneled segment. The total length of MB was 51.6 mm, the maximum halo thickness was 0.89 mm, the Max PB upstream of MB was 19.0%, and the maximum arterial compression was calculated as 37.6%.

operators from grossly identifying a tunneled coronary segment during the unroofing surgery. Detailed preoperative MB mapping by IVUS (see **Fig. 2**) can facilitate complete unroofing with minimum risk of surgical complications, which is crucial for successful outcomes.

SUMMARY

MB is a common congenital anomaly. Although the majority of patients with MB are asymptomatic, this anomaly can cause atherosclerotic plaque progression upstream from MB and hemodynamic disturbance owing to arterial systolic compression/diastolic restriction by MB, potentially leading to INOCA and adverse cardiac events, in a certain subset of patients. In MB patients with refractory angina, the optimal treatment strategy should be determined individually based on versatile anatomic and hemodynamical assessments with multidisciplinary diagnostic approaches. Among the currently available clinical imaging modalities, IVUS can play a unique role in this context by its ability to directly visualize the MB structure in a dynamic fashion.

CLINICS CARE POINTS

- Although MB is basically benign, be aware that it can contribute to cardiac adverse events such as angina and myocardial infarction.
- MB can be visualized by coronary CT or IVUS.
- When you find a significant MB, first consider introducing beta-blockers and nondihydropyridine calcium-channel blockers.
- When the patient with an MB is drug refractory, surgical unroofing may be effective rather than PCI or CABG.

DISCLOSURE

The authors have nothing to disclose.

ACKNOWLEDGMENTS

None.

REFERENCES

1. Humphries KH, Pu A, Gao M, et al. Angina with "normal" coronary arteries: sex differences in outcomes. Am Heart J 2008;155(2):375–81.
2. Patel MR, Dai D, Hernandez AF, et al. Prevalence and predictors of nonobstructive coronary artery disease identified with coronary angiography in contemporary clinical practice. Am Heart J 2014; 167(6):846–52.e2.
3. Lee BK, Lim HS, Fearon WF, et al. Invasive evaluation of patients with angina in the absence of obstructive coronary artery disease. Circulation 2015;131(12):1054–60.
4. Han SH, Bae JH, Holmes DR Jr, et al. Sex differences in atheroma burden and endothelial function in patients with early coronary atherosclerosis. Eur Heart J 2008;29(11):1359–69.
5. Siasos G, Sara JD, Zaromytidou M, et al. Local low shear stress and endothelial dysfunction in patients with nonobstructive coronary atherosclerosis. J Am Coll Cardiol 2018;71(19):2092–102.
6. Matta A, Nader V, Canitrot R, et al. Myocardial bridging is significantly associated to myocardial infarction with non-obstructive coronary arteries. Eur Heart J Acute Cardiovasc Care 2022;11(6): 501–7.
7. Ciçek D, Kalay N, Müderrisoğlu H. Incidence, clinical characteristics, and 4-year follow-up of patients with isolated myocardial bridge: a retrospective, single-center, epidemiologic, coronary arteriographic follow-up study in southern Turkey. Cardiovasc Revasc Med 2011;12(1):25–8.
8. Geiringer E. The mural coronary. Am Heart J 1951; 41(3):359–68.
9. Noble J, Bourassa MG, Petitclerc R, et al. Myocardial bridging and milking effect of the left anterior descending coronary artery: normal variant or obstruction? Am J Cardiol 1976;37(7):993–9.
10. Ishimori T, Raizner AE, Chahine RA, et al. Myocardial bridges in man: clinical correlations and angiographic accentuation with nitroglycerin. Cathet Cardiovasc Diagn 1977;3(1):59–65.
11. Lin S, Tremmel JA, Yamada R, et al. A novel stress echocardiography pattern for myocardial bridge with invasive structural and hemodynamic correlation. J Am Heart Assoc 2013;2(2):e000097.
12. Möhlenkamp S, Hort W, Ge J, et al. Update on myocardial bridging. Circulation 2002;106(20): 2616–22.
13. Tio RA, Van Gelder IC, Boonstra PW, et al. Myocardial bridging in a survivor of sudden cardiac near-death: role of intracoronary doppler flow measurements and angiography during dobutamine stress in the clinical evaluation. Heart 1997;77(3):280–2.
14. Kim PJ, Hur G, Kim SY, et al. Frequency of myocardial bridges and dynamic compression of epicardial coronary arteries: a comparison between computed tomography and invasive coronary angiography. Circulation 2009;119(10):1408–16.
15. Desseigne P, Tabib A, Loire R. Myocardial bridging on the left anterior descending coronary artery and

sudden death. Apropos of 19 cases with autopsy. Arch Mal Coeur Vaiss 1991;84(4):511–6 [in French].

16. Hashikata T, Honda Y, Wang H, et al. Impact of diastolic vessel restriction on quality of life in symptomatic myocardial bridging patients treated with surgical unroofing: preoperative assessments with intravascular ultrasound and coronary computed tomography angiography. Circ Cardiovasc Interv 2021;14(10):e011062.

17. Hongo Y, Tada H, Ito K, et al. Augmentation of vessel squeezing at coronary-myocardial bridge by nitroglycerin: study by quantitative coronary angiography and intravascular ultrasound. Am Heart J 1999;138(2 Pt 1):345–50.

18. Pargaonkar VS, Kimura T, Kameda R, et al. Invasive assessment of myocardial bridging in patients with angina and no obstructive coronary artery disease. EuroIntervention 2021;16(13):1070–8.

19. Rossi L, Dander B, Nidasio GP, et al. Myocardial bridges and ischemic heart disease. Eur Heart J 1980;1(4):239–45.

20. Juilliére Y, Berder V, Suty-Selton C, et al. Isolated myocardial bridges with angiographic milking of the left anterior descending coronary artery: a long-term follow-up study. Am Heart J 1995; 129(4):663–5.

21. Wymore P, Yedlicka JW, Garcia-Medina V, et al. The incidence of myocardial bridges in heart transplants. Cardiovasc Intervent Radiol 1989;12(4):202–6.

22. Tsujita K, Maehara A, Mintz GS, et al. Comparison of angiographic and intravascular ultrasonic detection of myocardial bridging of the left anterior descending coronary artery. Am J Cardiol 2008; 102(12):1608–13.

23. La Grutta L, Runza G, Lo Re G, et al. Prevalence of myocardial bridging and correlation with coronary atherosclerosis studied with 64-slice CT coronary angiography. Radiol Med 2009;114(7):1024–36.

24. Jeong YH, Kang MK, Park SR, et al. A head-to-head comparison between 64-slice multidetector computed tomographic and conventional coronary angiographies in measurement of myocardial bridge. Int J Cardiol 2010;143(3):243–8.

25. Liu G, Qu Y, Chen X, et al. Measurements of myocardial bridges on computed tomography predict presence of clinical symptoms and outcomes of adverse heart events: a retrospective study in a large population from China. Acta Radiol 2017; 58(9):1068–76.

26. Polacek P, Kralove H. Relation of myocardial bridges and loops on the coronary arteries to coronary occlusions. Am Heart J 1961;61:44–52.

27. Corban MT, Hung OY, Eshtehardi P, et al. Myocardial bridging: contemporary understanding of pathophysiology with implications for diagnostic and therapeutic strategies. J Am Coll Cardiol 2014;63(22):2346–55.

28. Hostiuc S, Negoi I, Rusu MC, et al. Myocardial bridging: a meta-analysis of prevalence. J Forensic Sci 2018;63(4):1176–85.

29. Ishii T, Hosoda Y, Osaka T, et al. The significance of myocardial bridge upon atherosclerosis in the left anterior descending coronary artery. J Pathol 1986;148(4):279–91.

30. Bayrak F, Degertekin M, Eroglu E, et al. Evaluation of myocardial bridges with 64-slice computed tomography coronary angiography. Acta Cardiol 2009;64(3):341–6.

31. Yamada R, Tremmel JA, Tanaka S, et al. Functional versus anatomic assessment of myocardial bridging by intravascular ultrasound: impact of arterial compression on proximal atherosclerotic plaque. J Am Heart Assoc 2016;5(4):e001735.

32. Iuchi A, Ishikawa Y, Akishima-Fukasawa Y, et al. Association of variance in anatomical elements of myocardial bridge with coronary atherosclerosis. Atherosclerosis 2013;227(1):153–8.

33. Yamada R, Turcott RG, Connolly AJ, et al. Histological characteristics of myocardial bridge with an ultrasonic echolucent band. Comparison between intravascular ultrasound and histology. Circ J 2014;78(2):502–4.

34. Liu H, Yamaguchi T. Computer modeling of fluid dynamics related to a myocardial bridge in a coronary artery. Biorheology 1999;36(5–6):373–90.

35. Herrmann J, Higano ST, Lenon RJ, et al. Myocardial bridging is associated with alteration in coronary vasoreactivity. Eur Heart J 2004;25(23):2134–42.

36. Ishikawa Y, Akasaka Y, Suzuki K, et al. Anatomic properties of myocardial bridge predisposing to myocardial infarction. Circulation 2009;120(5):376–83.

37. Kramer JR, Kitazume H, Proudfit WL, et al. Clinical significance of isolated coronary bridges: benign and frequent condition involving the left anterior descending artery. Am Heart J 1982;103(2):283–8.

38. Ge J, Erbel R, Görge G, et al. High wall shear stress proximal to myocardial bridging and atherosclerosis: intracoronary ultrasound and pressure measurements. Br Heart J 1995;73(5):462–5.

39. Navarro-Lopez F, Soler J, Magriña J, et al. Systolic compression of coronary artery in hypertrophic cardiomyopathy. Int J Cardiol 1986;12(3):309–20.

40. Rouleau JR, Roy L, Dumesnil JG, et al. Coronary vasodilator reserve impairment distal to systolic coronary artery compression in dogs. Cardiovasc Res 1983;17(2):96–105.

41. Pichard AD, Casanegra P, Marchant E, et al. Abnormal regional myocardial flow in myocardial bridging of the left anterior descending coronary artery. Am J Cardiol 1981;47(4):978–82.

42. Schwarz ER, Klues HG, vom Dahl J, et al. Functional, angiographic and intracoronary doppler flow characteristics in symptomatic patients with

myocardial bridging: effect of short-term intravenous beta-blocker medication. J Am Coll Cardiol 1996;27(7):1637–45.

43. Ge J, Jeremias A, Rupp A, et al. New signs characteristic of myocardial bridging demonstrated by intracoronary ultrasound and Doppler. Eur Heart J 1999;20(23):1707–16.

44. Cheng C, Tempel D, van Haperen R, et al. Atherosclerotic lesion size and vulnerability are determined by patterns of fluid shear stress. Circulation 2006;113(23):2744–53.

45. Ishii T, Asuwa N, Masuda S, et al. Atherosclerosis suppression in the left anterior descending coronary artery by the presence of a myocardial bridge: an ultrastructural study. Mod Pathol 1991;4(4): 424–31.

46. Kim JW, Seo HS, Na JO, et al. Myocardial bridging is related to endothelial dysfunction but not to plaque as assessed by intracoronary ultrasound. Heart 2008;94(6):765–9.

47. Ge J, Erbel R, Rupprecht HJ, et al. Comparison of intravascular ultrasound and angiography in the assessment of myocardial bridging. Circulation 1994;89(4):1725–32.

48. Cassar A, Chareonthaitawee P, Rihal CS, et al. Lack of correlation between noninvasive stress tests and invasive coronary vasomotor dysfunction in patients with nonobstructive coronary artery disease. Circ Cardiovasc Interv 2009;2(3):237–44.

49. Pargaonkar VS, Rogers IS, Su J, et al. Accuracy of a novel stress echocardiography pattern for myocardial bridging in patients with angina and no obstructive coronary artery disease - A retrospective and prospective cohort study. Int J Cardiol 2020;311:107–13.

50. Narula J, Chandrashekhar Y, Ahmadi A, et al. SCCT 2021 expert consensus document on coronary computed tomographic angiography: a report of the society of cardiovascular computed tomography. J Cardiovasc Comput Tomogr 2021;15(3): 192–217.

51. Knuuti J, Wijns W, Saraste A, et al. 2019 ESC guidelines for the diagnosis and management of chronic coronary syndromes. Eur Heart J 2020;41(3):407–77.

52. Forsdahl SH, Rogers IS, Schnittger I, et al. Myocardial bridges on coronary computed tomography angiography - correlation with intravascular ultrasound and fractional flow reserve. Circ J 2017; 81(12):1894–900.

53. Okamura A, Okura H, Iwai S, et al. Detection of myocardial bridge by optical coherence tomography. Int J Cardiovasc Imaging 2022. https://doi.org/10.1007/s10554-021-02497-5.

54. Nishimiya K, Matsumoto Y, Wang H, et al. Absence of adventitial vasa vasorum formation at the coronary segment with myocardial bridge - An optical coherence tomography study. Int J Cardiol 2018; 250:275–7.

55. Ohyama K, Matsumoto Y, Takanami K, et al. Coronary adventitial and perivascular adipose tissue inflammation in patients with vasospastic angina. J Am Coll Cardiol 2018;71(4):414–25.

56. Nair CK, Dang B, Heintz MH, et al. Myocardial bridges: effect of propranolol on systolic compression. Can J Cardiol 1986;2(4):218–21.

57. Alessandri N, Dei Giudici A, De Angelis S, et al. Efficacy of calcium channel blockers in the treatment of the myocardial bridging: a pilot study. Eur Rev Med Pharmacol Sci 2012;16(6):829–34.

58. Srinivasan M, Prasad A. Metal fatigue in myocardial bridges: stent fracture limits the efficacy of drug-eluting stents. J Invasive Cardiol 2011;23(6):E150–2.

59. Tsujita K, Maehara A, Mintz GS, et al. Serial intravascular ultrasound analysis of the impact of myocardial bridge on neointimal proliferation after coronary stenting in patients with acute myocardial infarction. J Interv Cardiol 2010;23(2):114–22.

60. Bockeria LA, Sukhanov SG, Orekhova EN, et al. Results of coronary artery bypass grafting in myocardial bridging of left anterior descending artery. J Card Surg 2013;28(3):218–21.

61. Cerrato E, Barbero U, D'Ascenzo F, et al. What is the optimal treatment for symptomatic patients with isolated coronary myocardial bridge? A systematic review and pooled analysis. J Cardiovasc Med (Hagerstown) 2017;18(10):758–70.

62. Boyd JH, Pargaonkar VS, Scoville DH, et al. Surgical unroofing of hemodynamically significant left anterior descending myocardial bridges. Ann Thorac Surg 2017;103(5):1443–50.

63. Wang H, Pargaonkar VS, Hironaka CE, et al. Off-pump minithoracotomy versus sternotomy for left anterior descending myocardial bridge unroofing. Ann Thorac Surg 2021;112(5):1474–82.

64. Maeda K, Schnittger I, Murphy DJ, et al. Surgical unroofing of hemodynamically significant myocardial bridges in a pediatric population. J Thorac Cardiovasc Surg 2018;156(4):1618–26.

Intravascular Imaging-Based Physiologic Assessment

Fumiyasu Seike, MD, PhD[a],*, Shinji Inaba, MD, PhD[a],
Kazunori Yasuda, PhD[b], Osamu Yamaguchi, MD, PhD[a]

KEYWORDS

- Intravascular ultrasound • Optical coherence tomography • Virtual fractional flow reserve
- Fluid dynamics

KEY POINTS

- Intravascular imaging-based virtual fractional flow reserve (FFR) measurement software calculated FFR with high accuracy (88% to 94%).
- The correlation between intracoronary virtual FFR and wire-based FFR was reportedly strong (0.69 to 0.89).
- The algorithms of intracoronary virtual FFR are based on basic fluid dynamics equations (mainly Poiseuille and Borda–Carnot equations) and original microvascular models (fixed velocity or calculating coronary flow reserve).
- The models and assumptions were based on the standard population (not independent patient data).

INTRODUCTION

Most interventional cardiologists rely on coronary angiography (CAG) to assess the severity of coronary artery disease and guide its treatment. However, the CAG has many known limitations since technically, it simply provides a foreshortened, shadowgraph, planar two-dimensional (2D) silhouette of the contrast-filled lumen. Intravascular imaging (IVI), including intravascular ultrasound (IVUS) and optical coherence tomography (OCT), is clinically useful for assessing the luminal size, lesion length, and plaque characteristics, as well as for evaluating stent deployment; however, it is not designed to estimate myocardial ischemia accurately.[1] With mounting evidence of fractional flow reserve (FFR) and the potential of fluid dynamics shown through FFR-computed tomography (CT),[2–6] several types of IVI-derived FFR (IVI-derived FFR) have been developed

and reported. This article explains the fundamentals of these methods and some future perspectives.

PRINCIPLES

Anatomic Factors and Myocardial Ischemia

Traditionally, CAG has been used to evaluate the severity of coronary lesions to determine the indication of percutaneous coronary intervention (PCI) or coronary artery bypass grafting for stable angina pectoris. However, there is a considerable mismatch reported between CAG severity and myocardial ischemia.[6] Although early IVUS studies showed reasonable correlations of minimum lumen area (MLA) measured by IVUS with results from physiologic assessments, limited diagnostic accuracies of IVUS-measured MLA in estimating myocardial ischemia have been reported in subsequent investigations with expanded patient populations.

---

[a] Department of Cardiology, Pulmonology, Hypertension & Nephrology, Ehime University Graduate School of Medicine, Shitsukawa, Toon, Ehime 791-0295, Japan; [b] Department of Mechanical Engineering, Ehime University Graduate School of Science and Engineering
* Corresponding author.
E-mail address: seike.fumiyasu.bn@ehime-u.ac.jp

Intervent Cardiol Clin 12 (2023) 289–298
https://doi.org/10.1016/j.iccl.2022.12.006
2211-7458/23/© 2023 Elsevier Inc. All rights reserved.

Intravascular imaging measurements and myocardial ischemia

There are three reasons that may account for the mismatch between anatomical measurements and myocardial ischemia[7].

1. Use of a single parameter

The standard luminal size of coronary artery depends on the location of the stenosis.[8,9] Thus, the MLA could not serve as the sole determinant of myocardial ischemia, independently of the lesion location. Moreover, longitudinal severity cannot be inferred from a single cross-sectional measurement, and indeed, coronary stenosis has many patterns with respect to axial disease extension. Thus, measurement of percent diameter or area stenosis (%AS) at the tightest site is also limited in estimating myocardial ischemia.[1] Combinations of anatomic parameters (ie, MLA + lesion length, % AS + lesion length) would improve the accuracy of detecting myocardial ischemia compared with the use of a single parameter.[1]

2. Parameter precision

Another technical reason for misevaluation may be attributable to the spatial resolution of the imaging modality.[10] The typical image resolution of CAG is 0.2 mm; thus, there may be large calculation errors for myocardial ischemia.[10] The spatial resolution of coronary CT angiography is 0.6 mm,[11] potentially requiring more estimation effort in accurately estimating myocardial ischemia. In contrast, IVI offers finer spatial resolutions, 0.1 mm in IVUS and 0.01 to 0.02 mm in OCT,[12] theoretically resulting in smaller errors in measurements compared with the other modalities.

3. Functional anatomical discordance

In the measurement of FFR as the gold standard in the diagnosis of myocardial ischemia, pressure loss is the primary determinant of the FFR value. According to fluid dynamics, friction loss and abrupt enhancement are the main causes of pressure loss in the coronary artery.[7] The Poiseuille equation can calculate friction loss due to viscosity:

$$\Delta P = \frac{8\pi\mu L}{As} \frac{An}{As} \times V$$

The Borda–Carnot equation can calculate pressure loss due to abrupt enhancement:

$$\Delta P = \frac{\rho}{2} \left(\frac{An}{As} - 1\right)^2 \times V^2$$

In both equations, L refers to the lesion length, μ refers to the blood viscosity, As refers to the lesion lumen area, An refers to the normal lumen area, ρ refers to the blood density, and V refers to the flow velocity. Therefore, although normal lumen area, MLA, and flow velocity are the main factors for pressure loss in coronary arteries, the pressure loss can be different even with equivalent structural factors, depending on the other factors. Regarding flow velocity, the velocities of the three coronary arteries are different from each other.[13] Consequently, even if the MLA or %AS values are the same, the severity of pressure loss (indicating FFR and myocardial ischemia) can be different in each case.

As described previously, many studies have tried to investigate the relationship between MLA determined by IVI and myocardial ischemia.[14–23] Table 1 shows the accuracy of MLA in the diagnosis of myocardial ischemia, which was 70% at most. The ranges of the cutoff values for IVUS- and OCT-MLA for myocardial ischemia were 2.4 to 4.0 mm² and 1.9 to 2.0 mm², respectively. Pooled analysis showed that the weighted overall mean MLA cutoff was 2.61 mm² in the non-left main (LM) trials and 5.35 mm² in the LM trials.[24] For non-LM lesions, the pooled sensitivity of MLA was 0.79 (95% confidence interval [CI] = 0.76 to 0.83) and specificity was 0.65 (95% CI = 0.62 to 0.67). Given the limited pooled accuracy of IVUS-MLA, its impact on clinical decision-making may not be sufficiently high, possibly leading to misclassification in up to 20% of lesions.[24]

Basic Theory of Calculating Intravascular Imaging-Based Fractional Flow Reserve

Table 2 summarizes the papers and data about intracoronary imaging virtual FFR software.[25–38] The key points of the algorithm in calculating virtual FFR are as follows.

1. Use of anatomical information

FFR-CT evaluates 3D coronary information as it is; however, 3D reconstruction and meshing generally require long calculation time and professional knowledge.[39] Thus, for almost all IVI-derived FFR (except for Ha and colleagues' method[31]), only lumen areas are used as anatomical information to reduce calculation time.

2. Fluid dynamics equation (Poiseuille and Borda–Carnot equations)

Virtual FFR software typically uses two types of equations to calculate pressure loss during

Table 1
Correlation and diagnostic accuracy between intracoronary imaging-derived minimum lumen area and myocardial ischemia

Publication	N	Reference	Image	Cut-off MLA, mm^2	R Value	Sensitivity	Specificity	Accuracy
Nishioka et al,[14] 1999	70	SPECT	IVUS	4.0	–	88%	90%	–
Takagi et al,[15] 1999	51	0.75	IVUS	3.0	0.786	83.0%	92.3%	–
Briguori et al,[16] 2001	53	0.75	IVUS	4.0	0.41	92%	56%	79%
Ben-Dor et al,[17] 2011	92	0.80	IVUS	3.2	0.34	69.2%	68.3%	70%
Kang et al,[18] 2011	236	0.80	IVUS	2.4	0.507	90%	60%	68%
Kang et al,[19] 2012	784	0.80	IVUS	2.4	0.481	83.2%	62.6%	68.5%
Koo et al,[20] 2011	267	0.80	IVUS	2.75	–	69%	65%	67%
Gonzalo et al,[21] 2012	47	0.80	OCT	1.95	0.520	82%	63%	72%
	47	0.80	IVUS	2.36	0.141	67%	65%	66%
Shiono et al,[22] 2012	62	0.75	OCT	1.91	0.75	93.5%	77.4%	85.4%
Waksman et al,[23] 2013	367	0.80	IVUS	3.07	0.55	64.0%	64.9%	–

Abbreviations: IVUS, intravascular ultrasound; MLA, minimum lumen area; OCT, optical coherence tomography.

hyperemia—fluid dynamics equations and myocardial circulation model (except for Ha and colleagues' method[31]). For instance, FFR-CT, the most commonly used virtual FFR software, uses the Navier–Stokes equations as the fluid dynamics equation and the lumped-parameter heart model as the assumed myocardial circulation model.[39]

The Navier–Stokes equation describes how the velocity, pressure, temperature, and density of a moving fluid are related. It can describe how the flow goes and behaves; however, except for simple fluid conditions, it is not applicable to most clinical cases. In the past, engineers made further approximations and simplifications to the equation until they had a group of solvable equations (eg, Poiseuille and Borda–Carnot equations). Recently, high-speed computers have been used to solve approximations for the equations using a variety of techniques. This area of study is called computational fluid dynamics (CFD). Unfortunately, however, it often requires long calculation and preparation time for daily practice, at least 2 to 3 h/case. Instead of the Navier–Stokes equation, simplified equations are used as fluid dynamics equations to reduce calculation time in IVI-based FFR. The Poiseuille and Borda–Carnot equations, or simplified equations based on these two equations, are used for basic fluid dynamics equations.

3. Hyperemic models (fixed coronary flow velocity or calculating coronary flow reserve [CFR])

Tu and colleagues developed several virtual FFR software such as the quantitative flow ratio (QFR) (CAG-based virtual FFR), ultrasonic flow ratio (UFR)[28] (IVUS-derived FFR), and OCT-based FFR (OFR).[33–37] UFR and OFR are now commercial software that can calculate virtual FFR in approximately 2 to 3 min (UFR) and 1 min (OFR), respectively. The virtual FFR values of UFR and OFR are obtained based on the basic fluid dynamics equations that calculate frictional losses along the entrance and throat of the stenosis and the inertial loss that is induced by the sudden expansion of flow as it emerges from the throat of the stenosis.[28] The reference lumen size, which is the healthy lumen size if there was no stenosis, is calculated based on the assumption that the healthy lumen will only decrease in size at the bifurcations following the bifurcation fractal laws. Considering the myocardial circulation model, 0.35 m/s of flow velocity is adapted for the UFR and OFR.[28,33–37]

The calculation of the virtual flow reserve (VFR) is based on a lumped-parameter model of the blood flow through a stenosed artery as the hyperemic model[29] Fig. 1. VFR adapts equations based on the Poiseuille and Borda–Carnot equations as epicardial artery resistance. In this model, the blood flow (Q), driven by the difference between the mean aortic and venous pressures, Pav = Pa–Pv, is limited by the total flow resistance of the branch, which is composed of three resistance elements, RT = Rs + Re + Rmv, where Rs is the blood flow resistance of the stenotic segment, Re is the blood flow resistance of the

Table 2
Correlations and accuracy of intracoronary imaging-derived fractional flow reserve for wire-based fractional flow reserve

Modality	Authors, Year	Pt (Vessels)	Correlation	Fluid Dynamics Equations	Circulation Model	Accuracy	AUC
IVUS	Takayama & Hodgson,[25] 2001	13(14)	0.95	Poiseuille and Borda–Carnot equations	0.5 m/s	–	–
	Seike et al,[26] 2018	48(50)	0.78	Poiseuille and Borda–Carnot equations	SFR	–	–
	Bezerra et al,[27] 2019	24(34)	0.79	0.89	0.92	0.91	0.93
	Yu et al,[28] 2021	94(167)	0.87	0.91	0.35 m/s	0.92	0.97
OCT	Guagliumi et al,[29] 2013	21(21)	0.81	Based on the Poiseuille and Borda–Carnot equations	Lumped model	–	–
	Zafar et al,[30] 2014	20(26)	0.69	–	–	–	–
	Ha et al,[31] 2016	92(92)	0.72	Navier–Stokes equations	TIMI flame count	0.88	0.93
	Seike et al,[32] 2017	31(31)	0.89	Poiseuille and Borda–Carnot equation	SFR	–	–
	Lee et al,[33] 2017	13(17)	0.66	Basic fluid dynamics equation	0.35 m/s	0.94	–
	Yu et al,[34] 2019	118(125)	0.70	Basic fluid dynamics equation	0.35 m/s	0.90	0.93
	Gutierrez et al,[35] 2020	60(76)	0.83	Basic fluid dynamics equation	0.35 m/s	0.93	0.95
	Huang et al,[36] 2020	181(212)	0.87	Basic fluid dynamics equation	0.35 m/s	0.92	0.97
	Emori et al,[37] 2020	103(103)	0.84	Basic fluid dynamics equation	0.35 m/s	–	–
	Cha et al,[38] 2020	25	0.85	Machine learning	Machine learning	0.95	0.98

Abbreviations: AUC, area under the curve; IVUS, intravascular ultrasound; OCT, optical coherence tomography; Pt, patients; Sens., sensitivity; Spec, specificity.

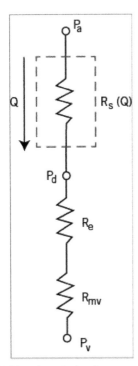

Fig. 1. VFR (virtual optical coherence tomography-derived FFR) adapts the Poiseuille and Borda–Carnot equations, which are used for epicardial artery resistance as the Ohm model (28). In this model, the blood flow (Q), driven by the difference between the mean aortic and venous pressures, Pav = Pa – Pv, is limited by the total flow resistance of the branch, which is composed of three resistance elements, RT = Rs + Re + Rmv, where Rs is the blood flow resistance of the stenotic segment, Re is the blood flow resistance of vessel length outside the lesion, and Rmv is the microvascular resistance under maximal hyperemia (28).

vessel length outside the lesion, and Rmv is the microvascular resistance under maximal hyperemia.[29] The widths of the branches are shown in an ordinate scale, and the flow volume in the main artery is reduced according to the size of the side branch (Fig. 2B). The Functional Diagnosis of Coronary Stenosis (FUSION) Study[40] is investigating the reliability of the VFR model through the validation of the diagnostic performance of VFR by comparing it against a reference standard FFR ClinicalTrials.gov number, NCT04356027).

Seike and colleagues[26,32] developed a virtual FFR model for IVUS and OCT, wherein the Poiseuille and Borda–Carnot equations are used directly for epicardial artery resistance. The stenotic flow reserve model (SFR) developed by Gould and colleagues[41] was modified as a microvascular circulation model. SFR calculates the virtual CFR using a mathematical circulation

model of microvascular pressure loss by subtracting pressure loss due to epicardial stenosis from aortic pressure (Fig. 2). The SFR concept is similar to the lumped-parameter model, such that both methods calculate the balance of pressure loss between microvascular resistance and epicardial coronary stenosis. The physiological assumptions were modified as follows: changing flow velocities according to coronary arteries and changing flow velocity and blood pressure between the diastolic and systolic phases.

Ha and colleagues[31] investigated the virtual FFR method for the left anterior descending artery by using the CFD model. Flow velocity was calculated based on the thrombolysis in myocardial infarction (TIMI) frame count. However, the calculation and preparation of 3D reconstruction and meshing require a long calculation time; thus, it would be difficult to use these as the standard during daily catheterization practice. These types of CFD-based coronary flow assessment may help investigate the mechanisms of atherosclerosis, plaque rupture, and thrombus formations.

OCT measurement-based machine learning FFR has also been reported,[38] which could be used to simultaneously acquire both imaging and functional information during one single diagnostic procedure. It is highly expected that machine-learning-based methods would further advance the development of clinically useful virtual FFR software in the near future.

CORRELATIONS AND DIAGNOSTIC ACCURACY

The correlation and diagnostic accuracy of IVI-derived FFR for myocardial ischemia are shown in Table 2.[25–38] In IVUS-derived FFR, the correlations between and wire-based FFR of 0.78 to 0.95, areas under the curve of 0.93 to 0.97, and accuracies of 0.91 to 0.97 have been shown. The correlations of OCT-derived FFR have also been reported as 0.69 to 0.89, areas under the curve as 0.93 to 0.97, and accuracies as 0.88 to 0.94. Of note, coronary revascularization guided by the instantaneous wave-free ratio (iFR) has been shown to be noninferior to revascularization guided by FFR with respect to the risk of major adverse cardiac events.[42,43] A meta-analysis[44] showed that iFR significantly correlates with standard FFR (0.798 [0.78 to 0.82], $P < 0.001$) along with a good diagnostic performance in identifying FFR-positive myocardial ischemia (area under the curve = 0.88 [0.86 to 0.90], $P < 0.001$). Compared with the above data shown for iFR as referenced to standard

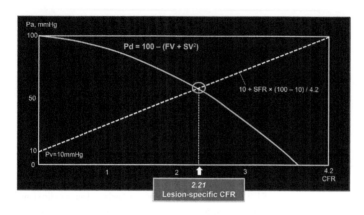

Fig. 2. The modified SFR model was used to calculate virtual fractional flow reserve (FFR). The SFR model, which was developed by Gould et al. (40), was modified as a microvascular circulation model. SFR calculates virtual coronary flow reserve using a mathematical circulation model of microvascular pressure loss by subtracting pressure loss due to epicardial stenosis from aortic pressure. A linear function of flow completely describes the pressure difference across the downstream myocardial bed during hyperemia. SFR occurs at the point where the quadratic function describing the stenosis intersects the linear function describing the myocardial bed (100 mm Hg) and venous or backpressure (10 mm Hg) are used (To calculate CFR only, systolic blood pressure 120 mmHg, diastolic blood pressure 60 mmHg, and mean blood pressure 80 mmHg are adapted to calculate FFR). Normal CFR = 4.2, 2.0 in the absence of a stenosis for the diastolic and systolic phases, respectively.

FFR, the efficacy of IVI-derived FFR is at the same level. One caution, however, is that virtual FFR studies excluded relatively complex lesions/vessels, diffuse coronary artery stenosis, ostial lesion, left ventricular hypertrophy, and valvular heart disease. Therefore, further studies are required for IVI-derived FFR to be validated in complex lesion/patient subsets.

LIMITATIONS

The virtual FFR algorithm requires many parameters including blood viscosity and density, blood pressure, and resting/hyperemic coronary flow velocity for each epicardial artery. These parameters are assumed based on typical group behaviors, and not on individual patients' heart and coronary conditions. Detailed limitations of these assumptions are explained below.

Theoretically, the Poiseuille equation should be adapted for a Newtonian fluid (steady laminar flow with full development), whereas the Borda–Carnot equation should be adapted for fluid with no friction (steady and having constant density). Blood is a non-Newtonian fluid; moreover, blood flow does not develop fully in the coronary artery because of its length, curvature, and branches. The Borda–Carnot and Poiseuille equations can be adjusted to calculate for pressure loss; however, these equations do not completely work in coronary arteries. Blood pressure under hyperemia, which may vary depending on the patients, are adapted for common patients. Blood density and viscosity could also vary with a normal range, respectively.

Pressure loss depends mainly on flow volume according to the fluid dynamics equations. Flow

volume is assumed depending on the: (1) assumed resting flow velocity, (2) theoretical maximal CFR, and (3) normal reference area. The resting flow velocity of coronary arteries can vary depending on the patients.[13] The CFR is dependent on the combined effects of epicardial coronary stenosis and microvascular dysfunction, thereby resulting in impaired CFR reflecting the presence of microvascular dysfunction in the absence of obstructive coronary artery.[45] Thus, it is difficult to evaluate microvascular dysfunction and theoretical maximal CFR by using intracoronary imaging only. Finally, the "normal" lumen area of each segment may not be truly normal due to the diffuse nature of atherosclerosis and vessel remodeling whereas each algorithm tested in the literature assumed that it is.

FUTURE PERSPECTIVES

From a practical perspective, IVI-derived FFR software should be integrated in imaging systems in catheterization laboratories because it would shorten the preparation and calculation time for virtual FFR. If the accuracy of the VFR method is successfully validated in the ongoing prospective multi-center FUSION study,[40] this software may become a frontrunner in the IVI-derived FFR methods in the clinical arena.

To date, there are three major types of virtual FFR software: (1) CT-derived FFR,[2–6] (2) angiography-derived FFR,[46–49] and (3) IVI (IVUS and OCT)-derived FFR. The CT-derived FFR and angiography-derived FFR have already been introduced in clinical practice. Since these two techniques are less invasive, IVI-derived FFR would be limited for the sole use of pre-PCI physiological evaluation. However, it may play a unique role at PCI guidance and optimization, potentially allowing comprehensive and time/cost-saving assessment of both anatomical and physiological lesion properties using a single diagnostic device. Table 3 summarizes the additional values of IVI-derived FFR on image-guided PCI.

1. Pre-evaluation

The 2021 American College of Cardiology/American Heart Association/Society for Cardiovascular Angiography and Interventions (ACC/AHA/SCAI) Guideline for Coronary Artery Revascularization[50] recommends intracoronary imaging-guided PCI for complex lesions. When IVUS or OCT is used for PCI guidance, physiological assessment with IVI-derived FFR, rather than adding wire-based FFR, may reduce the total cost of CAG and PCI. IVI-derived FFR may also be useful when other imaging-derived FFR methods suffer difficulty in accurately evaluating lumen size because of complex lesion morphology, such as severe calcifications or bifurcation lesions. Although it has been reported that FFR-CT could provide superior diagnostic performance overall to standard coronary CT angiography interpretation alone in patients/vessels with significant calcification,[51] the calculation of FFR-CT values could theoretically be affected in severely calcified lesions. Bifurcation lesions could also be challenging for accurate evaluation with CAG alone. Huang and colleagues[36] reported that IVI-derived FFR (OFR) was superior to angiography-derived FFR (QFR) and was better than conventional morphological parameters in determining the physiological significance of coronary stenosis.

2. PCI support

In daily clinical practice, repeated FFR measurements for PCI treatment of tandem lesions are time-consuming and costly. In a case series of OCT-derived FFR, Okuya and colleagues[52] reported that their method could evaluate FFR at each lesion level for tandem lesions without any cross talk. This approach may enable the independent evaluation of the severity of each lesion and pressure loss, unaffected by another stenosis in the same vessel, thereby allowing precise PCI planning and evaluation with physiological assessment. Fig. 3 is a representative PCI case supported by IVI-derived FFR. The DEFINE GPS (Distal Evaluation of Functional performance with Intravascular sensors to assess the Narrowing Effect: Guided Physiologic Stenting, ClinicalTrials.gov number, NCT04451044)[53] study was the first to use iFR in conjunction with the Philips Image-Guided Co-registration System (SyncVision) for the evaluation of PCI guidance and optimization of treatment outcomes, focusing on identifying the locations of physiologically significant lesions. The lesion-level physiological assessment is now gaining increasing attention as a key to successful PCI, where IVI-derived FFR may also play a unique role with its ability to assess the functional severity of each lesion combined with detailed structural information.

3. Post-PCI evaluation

Greater stent expansion and less stent-edge plaque burden maximize the probability of stent patency.[1] However, the cut-off value of minimum stent area to best predict subsequent in-stent restenosis varies depending on the lesion location in coronary arteries.[54] In this context, virtual in-stent FFR would help in the assessment of residual stenosis from the functional perspective. It has been reported that post-PCI FFR values have an impact on clinical outcomes,[55,56] and suboptimal virtual FFR values after PCI can result from three mechanisms.[57] First, initially unappreciated, unmasked tandem lesions occasionally increase gradients dramatically after

Table 3
Additional values of intracoronary imaging-derived fractional flow reserve on image-guided percutaneous coronary intervention

Pre PCI	Vessel-level physiological assessment
	Lesion-level physiological assessment
During PCI	Post-stenting FFR estimation (virtual stenting)
	Assistance in determining the segment to be treated
Post-PCI	Vessel-level post-stenting physiological assessment
	Stented-segment physiological assessment
	Nonculprit vessel assessment
	Nonculprit lesion assessment

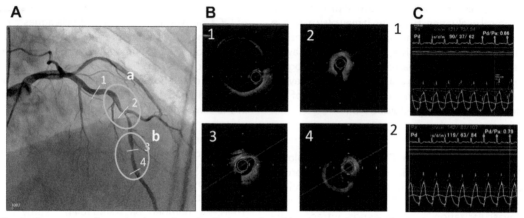

Fig. 3. Coronary angiography showed tandem lesion in the mid segment of the left descending artery (A). Optical coherence tomography showed minimum lumen area 0.83 mm^2 at the proximal portion, 1.02 mm^2 at the distal stenosis (B). Optical coherence tomography (OCT)-derived FFR (fractional flow reserve) can calculate each lesion severity independently without any flow interaction. OCT-derived FFR for vessel, proximal lesion, distal lesion were calculated as 0.64, 0.67 and 0.77, respectively. Vessel wire-based FFR was 0.66 (C1). Stent was deployed at the proximal stenosis according to the OCT-derived FFR, after stenting wire-based FFR was 0.79 (C2). OCT-derived FFR for distal could evaluated the distal lesion physiological severity precisely before stenting.

the PCI of the primary stenosis. Second, stent implantation causes a gradient as shown by longitudinal observations. Third, diffuse diseases frequently coexist with focal lesions and remain untreated after PCI. IVI with IVI-derived FFR at post-PCI may offer comprehensive and time/cost-saving assessment of both the anatomical and physiological properties of the treated lesion using a single diagnostic device. Further studies are warranted to validate the clinical efficacy of this novel approach.

CLINICS CARE POINTS

- Intravascular imaging-based virtual fractional flow reserve (FFR) measurement software calculated FFR with high accuracy and correlation.

- The algorithms of intracoronary virtual FFR are based on basic fluid dynamics equations and original microvascular models.

- It may play a unique role at PCI guidance and optimization, potentially allowing comprehensive and time/cost-saving assessment of both anatomical and physiological lesion properties using a single diagnostic device.

DISCLOSURE

Dr F. Seike received lecture fee from Abbott Vascular.

REFERENCES

1. Mintz GS, Guagliumi G. Intravascular imaging in coronary artery disease. Lancet 2017;390(10096):793–809.
2. Celeng C, Leiner T, Maurovich-Horvat P, et al. Anatomical and Functional Computed Tomography for Diagnosing Hemodynamically Significant Coronary Artery Disease: A Meta-Analysis. JACC Cardiovasc Imaging 2019;12(7 Pt 2):1316–25.
3. Driessen RS, Danad I, Stuijfzand WJ, et al. Comparison of Coronary Computed Tomography Angiography, Fractional Flow Reserve, and Perfusion Imaging for Ischemia Diagnosis. J Am Coll Cardiol 2019;73(2):161–73.
4. Fairbairn TA, Nieman K, Akasaka T, et al. Real-world clinical utility and impact on clinical decision-making of coronary computed tomography angiography-derived fractional flow reserve: lessons from the ADVANCE Registry. Eur Heart J 2018;39(41):3701–11.
5. Douglas PS, Pontone G, Hlatky MA, et al. Clinical outcomes of fractional flow reserve by computed tomographic angiography-guided diagnostic strategies vs. usual care in patients with suspected coronary artery disease: the prospective longitudinal trial of FFR(CT): outcome and resource impacts study. Eur Heart J 2015;36(47):3359–67.
6. Park SJ, Kang SJ, Ahn JM, et al. Visual-functional mismatch between coronary angiography and fractional flow reserve. JACC Cardiovasc Interv 2012;5(10):1029–36.
7. Johnson NP, Kirkeeide RL, Gould KL. Coronary anatomy to predict physiology: fundamental limits. Circ Cardiovasc Imaging 2013;6(5):817–32.
8. Dodge JT Jr, Brown BG, Bolson EL, et al. Lumen diameter of normal human coronary arteries.

Influence of age, sex, anatomic variation, and left ventricular hypertrophy or dilation. Circulation 1992;86(1):232–46.

9. Javier SP, Mintz GS, Popma JJ, et al. Intravascular ultrasound assessment of the magnitude and mechanism of coronary artery and lumen tapering. Am J Cardiol 1995;75(2):177–80.

10. Keane D, Haase J, Slager CJ, et al. Comparative validation of quantitative coronary angiography systems. Results and implications from a multi-center study using a standardized approach. Circulation 1995;91(8):2174–83.

11. Voros S, Rinehart S, Qian Z, et al. Coronary atherosclerosis imaging by coronary CT angiography: current status, correlation with intravascular interrogation and meta-analysis. JACC Cardiovasc Imaging 2011;4(5):537–48.

12. Bezerra HG, Costa MA, Guagliumi G, et al. Intracoronary optical coherence tomography: a comprehensive review clinical and research applications. JACC Cardiovasc Interv 2009;2(11):1035–46.

13. Wieneke H, Haude M, Ge J, et al. Corrected coronary flow velocity reserve: a new concept for assessing coronary perfusion. J Am Coll Cardiol 2000;35(7):1713–20.

14. Nishioka T, Amanullah AM, Luo H, et al. Clinical validation of intravascular ultrasound imaging for assessment of coronary stenosis severity: comparison with stress myocardial perfusion imaging. J Am Coll Cardiol 1999;33(7):1870–8.

15. Takagi A, Tsurumi Y, Ishii Y, et al. Clinical potential of intravascular ultrasound for physiological assessment of coronary stenosis: relationship between quantitative ultrasound tomography and pressure-derived fractional flow reserve. Circulation 1999;100(3):250–5.

16. Briguori C, Anzuini A, Airoldi F, et al. Intravascular ultrasound criteria for the assessment of the functional significance of intermediate coronary artery stenoses and comparison with fractional flow reserve. Am J Cardiol 2001;87(2):136–41.

17. Ben-Dor I, Torguson R, Gaglia MA Jr, et al. Correlation between fractional flow reserve and intravascular ultrasound lumen area in intermediate coronary artery stenosis. EuroIntervention 2011;7(2):225–33.

18. Kang SJ, Lee JY, Ahn JM, et al. Validation of intravascular ultrasound-derived parameters with fractional flow reserve for assessment of coronary stenosis severity. Circ Cardiovasc Interv 2011;4(1):65–71.

19. Kang SJ, Ahn JM, Song H, et al. Usefulness of minimal luminal coronary area determined by intravascular ultrasound to predict functional significance in stable and unstable angina pectoris. Am J Cardiol 2012;109(7):947–53.

20. Koo BK, Yang HM, Doh JH, et al. Optimal intravascular ultrasound criteria and their accuracy for defining the functional significance of intermediate coronary stenoses of different locations. JACC Cardiovasc Interv 2011;4(7):803–11.

21. Gonzalo N, Escaned J, Alfonso F, et al. Morphometric assessment of coronary stenosis relevance with optical coherence tomography: a comparison with fractional flow reserve and intravascular ultrasound. J Am Coll Cardiol 2012;59(12):1080–9.

22. Shiono Y, Kitabata H, Kubo T, et al. Optical coherence tomography-derived anatomical criteria for functionally significant coronary stenosis assessed by fractional flow reserve. Circ J 2012;76(9):2218–25.

23. Waksman R, Legutko J, Singh J, et al. FIRST: Fractional Flow Reserve and Intravascular Ultrasound Relationship Study. J Am Coll Cardiol 2013;61(9):917–23.

24. Nascimento BR, de Sousa MR, Koo BK, et al. Diagnostic accuracy of intravascular ultrasound-derived minimal lumen area compared with fractional flow reserve—meta-analysis: pooled accuracy of IVUS luminal area versus FFR. Catheter Cardiovasc Interv 2014;84(3):377–85.

25. Takayama T, Hodgson JM. Prediction of the physiologic severity of coronary lesions using 3D IVUS: validation by direct coronary pressure measurements. Catheter Cardiovasc Interv 2001;53(1):48–55.

26. Seike F, Uetani T, Nishimura K, et al. Intravascular Ultrasound-Derived Virtual Fractional Flow Reserve for the Assessment of Myocardial Ischemia. Circ J 2018;82(3):815–23.

27. Bezerra CG, Hideo-Kajita A, Bulant CA, et al. Coronary fractional flow reserve derived from intravascular ultrasound imaging: Validation of a new computational method of fusion between anatomy and physiology. Catheter Cardiovasc Interv 2019;93(2):266–74.

28. Yu W, Tanigaki T, Ding D, et al. Accuracy of Intravascular Ultrasound-Based Fractional Flow Reserve in Identifying Hemodynamic Significance of Coronary Stenosis. Circ Cardiovasc Interv 2021;14(2):e009840.

29. Guagliumi G, Sirbu V, Petroff C, et al. Volumetric assessment of lesion severity with optical coherence tomography: relationship with fractional flow. EuroIntervention 2013;8(10):1172–81.

30. Zafar H, Sharif F, Leahy MJ. Feasibility of intracoronary frequency domain optical coherence tomography derived fractional flow reserve for the assessment of coronary artery stenosis. Int Heart J 2014;55:307–11.

31. Ha J, Kim JS, Lim J, et al. Assessing computational fractional flow reserve from optical coherence tomography in patients with intermediate coronary stenosis in the left anterior descending artery. Circ Cardiovasc Interv 2016;9:e003613.

32. Seike F, Uetani T, Nishimura K, et al. Intracoronary optical coherence tomography-derived virtual fractional flow reserve for the assessment of coronary artery disease. Am J Cardiol 2017;120:1772–9.

33. Lee KE, Lee SH, Shin ES, et al. A vessel length-based method to compute coronary fractional flow reserve from optical coherence tomography images. Biomed Eng Online 2017;16:83.

34. Yu W, Huang J, Jia D, et al. Diagnostic accuracy of intracoronary optical coherence tomography-derived fractional flow reserve for assessment of coronary stenosis severity. EuroIntervention 2019; 15:189–97.

35. Gutiérrez-Chico JL, Chen Y, Yu W, et al. Diagnostic accuracy and reproducibility of optical flow ratio for functional evaluation of coronary stenosis in a prospective series. Cardiol J 2020;27(4):350–61.

36. Huang J, Emori H, Ding D, et al. Diagnostic performance of intracoronary optical coherence tomography-based versus angiography-based fractional flow reserve for the evaluation of coronary lesions. EuroIntervention 2020;16(7):568–76.

37. Emori H, Kubo T, Shiono Y, et al. Comparison of Optical Flow Ratio and Fractional Flow Ratio in Stent-Treated Arteries Immediately After Percutaneous Coronary Intervention. Circ J 2020;84(12):2253–8.

38. Cha JJ, Son TD, Ha J, et al. Optical coherence tomography-based machine learning for predicting fractional flow reserve in intermediate coronary stenosis: a feasibility study. Sci Rep 2020;10(1):20421.

39. Taylor CA, Fonte TA, Min JK. Computational fluid dynamics applied to cardiac computed tomography for noninvasive quantification of fractional flow reserve: scientific basis. J Am Coll Cardiol 2013;61(22):2233–41.

40. Available at: https://clinicaltrials.gov/ct2/show/NCT04356027.

41. Gould KL, Kelley KO, Bolson EL. Experimental validation of quantitative coronary arteriography for determining pressure-flow characteristics of coronary stenosis. Circulation 1982;66(5):930–7.

42. Davies JE, Sen S, Dehbi HM, et al. Use of the Instantaneous Wave-free Ratio or Fractional Flow Reserve in PCI. N Engl J Med 2017;376(19):1824–34.

43. Gotberg M, Christiansen EH, Gudmundsdottir IJ, et al. iFR-SWEDEHEART Investigators. Instantaneous Wave-free Ratio versus Fractional Flow Reserve to Guide PCI. N Engl J Med 2017;376(19):1813–23.

44. De Rosa S, Polimeni A, Petraco R, et al. Diagnostic Performance of the Instantaneous Wave-Free Ratio: Comparison With Fractional Flow Reserve. Circ Cardiovasc Interv 2018;11(1):e004613.

45. Hirata K, Amudha K, Elina R, et al. Measurement of coronary vasomotor function: getting to the heart of the matter in cardiovascular research. Clin Sci (Lond) 2004;107(5):449–60.

46. Kornowski R, Lavi I, Pellicano M, et al. Fractional Flow Reserve Derived From Routine Coronary Angiograms. J Am Coll Cardiol 2016;68(20):2235–7.

47. Witberg G, De Bruyne B, Fearon WF, et al. Diagnostic Performance of Angiogram-Derived Fractional Flow Reserve: A Pooled Analysis of 5 Prospective Cohort Studies. JACC Cardiovasc Interv 2020;13(4):488–97.

48. Westra J, Andersen BK, Campo G, et al. Diagnostic Performance of In-Procedure Angiography-Derived Quantitative Flow Reserve Compared with Pressure-Derived Fractional Flow Reserve: The FAVOR II Europe-Japan Study. J Am Heart Assoc 2018;7(14):e009603.

49. Masdjedi K, van Zandvoort LJC, Balbi MM, et al. Validation of a three-dimensional quantitative coronary angiography-based software to calculate fractional flow reserve: the FAST study. EuroIntervention 2020; 16(7):591–9.

50. Lawton JS, Tamis-Holland JE, Bangalore S, et al. 2021 ACC/AHA/SCAI Guideline for Coronary Artery Revascularization: Executive Summary: A Report of the American College of Cardiology/American Heart Association Joint Committee on Clinical Practice Guidelines. J Am Coll Cardiol 2022;79(2):197–215.

51. Norgaard BL, Gaur S, Leipsic J, et al. Influence of Coronary Calcification on the Diagnostic Performance of CT Angiography Derived FFR in Coronary Artery Disease: A Substudy of the NXT Trial. JACC Cardiovasc Imaging. 2015;8(9):1045-1055. doi: .

52. Okuya Y, Seike F, Yoneda K, et al. Functional assessment of tandem coronary artery stenosis by intracoronary optical coherence tomography-derived virtual fractional flow reserve: a case series. Eur Heart J Case Rep 2019;3(2):ytz087.

53. Available at: https://clinicaltrials.gov/ct2/show/NCT04451044.

54. Kang SJ, Ahn JM, Song H, et al. Comprehensive intravascular ultrasound assessment of stent area and its impact on restenosis and adverse cardiac events in 403 patients with unprotected left main disease. Circ Cardiovasc Interv 2011;4(6):562–9.

55. Doh JH, Nam CW, Koo BK, et al. Clinical Relevance of Poststent Fractional Flow Reserve After Drug-Eluting Stent Implantation. J Invasive Cardiol 2015;27(8):346–51.

56. Nam CW, Hur SH, Cho YK, et al. Relation of fractional flow reserve after drug-eluting stent implantation to one-year outcomes. Am J Cardiol 2011; 107(12):1763–7.

57. Tonino PA, Johnson NP. Why Is Fractional Flow Reserve After Percutaneous Coronary Intervention Not Always 1.0? JACC Cardiovasc Interv 2016;9(10):1032–5.

Printed and bound by CPI Group (UK) Ltd, Croydon, CR0 4YY

03/10/2024

01040365-0013